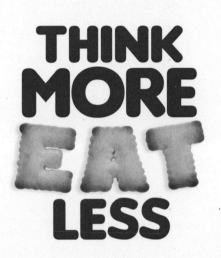

THINK MORE EAT LESS

THINK
MORE
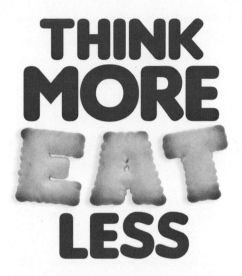
EAT
LESS

Use Your Mind to
Change Your Body

JANET THOMSON MSc

HAY HOUSE

Australia • Canada • Hong Kong • India
South Africa • United Kingdom • United States

First published and distributed in the United Kingdom by:
Hay House UK Ltd, 292B Kensal Rd, London W10 5BE.
Tel.: (44) 20 8962 1230; Fax: (44) 20 8962 1239.
www.hayhouse.co.uk

Published and distributed in the United States of America by:
Hay House, Inc., PO Box 5100, Carlsbad, CA 92018-5100.
Tel.: (1) 760 431 7695 or (800) 654 5126; Fax: (1) 760 431 6948 or (800) 650 5115.
www.hayhouse.com

Published and distributed in Australia by:
Hay House Australia Ltd, 18/36 Ralph St, Alexandria NSW 2015.
Tel.: (61) 2 9669 4299; Fax: (61) 2 9669 4144.
www.hayhouse.com.au

Published and distributed in the Republic of South Africa by:
Hay House SA (Pty), Ltd, PO Box 990, Witkoppen 2068.
Tel./Fax: (27) 11 467 8904. www.hayhouse.co.za

Published and distributed in India by:
Hay House Publishers India, Muskaan Complex, Plot No.3, B-2,
Vasant Kunj, New Delhi – 110 070. Tel.: (91) 11 4176 1620; Fax: (91) 11 4176 1630.
www.hayhouse.co.in

Distributed in Canada by:
Raincoast, 9050 Shaughnessy St, Vancouver, BC V6P 6E5.
Tel.: (1) 604 323 7100; Fax: (1) 604 323 2600

Text © Janet Thomson, 2012

Mabel illustrations © Luke Martin, 2011

The information given in this book should not be treated as a substitute for professional medical advice; always consult a medical practitioner. Any use of information in this book is at the reader's discretion and risk. Neither the author nor the publisher can be held responsible for any loss, claim or damage arising out of the use, or misuse, or the suggestions made or the failure to take medical advice. A catalogue record for this book is available from the British Library.

ISBN: 978-1-84850-712-8

Printed and bound in Great Britain by TJ International, Padstow, Cornwall.

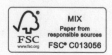

MIX
Paper from
responsible sources
FSC® C013056

CONTENTS

Contents

Contents

Contents

ACKNOWLEDGEMENTS

For me this is perhaps the most significant page in this book. You cannot underestimate the value of a strong supportive network when striving to achieve a goal. What you are about to read is the result of 25 years of working with clients to help them lose weight. There have been many highs and lows along the way, as I have learnt and refined my craft so that I can share it with you now. There are people in my life who have truly gone out of their way to support me in achieving my vision of transforming as many minds and bodies as possible. In no particular order, Nicole Barber Lane, Deirdre Randall, Ramona Barretto, Nikki Malone, Caroline Sheridan, Clare Pykett, Louise and Stephen Fordham, Joy and Gerry Martin, Sophie Thornton and Pam McLoughlin have all extended love and friendship to me above and beyond the call of duty, and for that I am truly grateful.

I would like to also express my deep appreciation to Michelle Pilley, Carolyn Thorne, Jo Burgess and the team at Hay House. My vision was for a completely different 'diet' book, bringing together mind and body, and they totally supported this vision. Thank you also to Luke Martin for the wonderful drawings of Mabel.

And lastly thank you to Mabel – you know who you are. Your true story will inspire, so thanks for sharing.

INTRODUCTION

Let's get straight down to it. You are fat and you want to be slim. Maybe you are a few kilos overweight, or perhaps you are obese – either way, I will help you to help yourself. I won't do it for you, though – and believe me, you'll be grateful for that, because the sense of achievement you are going to get once *you* have changed how you *think and feel, and look*, is priceless. Now that you've decided to take this step, the feeling is coming your way!

The title of this book is *Think More, Eat Less*, but it could just as easily have been *Eat Less and Think Differently* or *Eat Less, Think More*. In a way, all of these titles imply that you are *not thinking*, but in fact, you are *never* not thinking! You may let any old thought come and go, without actually controlling it, but you are *always thinking*. Your thoughts are the way that you communicate with yourself, so you are never not communicating with *yourself*. Let me say that again:

You are never not communicating with yourself.

So how good is your communication with *you*? We spend so much time thinking about how we come across to other people, but have you wondered how you'd come across to *yourself*? If you'd just met you, what would your opinion be of how well you look after your body? What score would you give yourself out of 10 in that category? I'm guessing it wouldn't be top of the class, otherwise you wouldn't be overweight, *but* (don't worry, it's a 'good' but!) you *can* be top of the class – in fact you can be top of the school.

Once you've read this book, you can be so good that you become the teacher and inspire other people, because you'll probably want to share what you've learnt with everyone you know who can benefit from it. Not only will *you* feel good, but you will help *other people*, too, and that's one of the most rewarding feelings in the world. So, are you hungry for it? Pardon the pun, but as you'll discover, a sense of humour is very helpful for instigating change. If it's fun, it's easier!

I'm guessing that some aspects of your communication with *you* are already pretty good. I'll bet, for instance, that you are great at communicating excuses, at procrastinating, and at telling yourself what you 'should' do and then creating a thousand reasons why you *can't* or *don't* do it! If you're nodding as you read this, then I'm probably right! That's a good start. At least we're agreed that on some level you are already a good communicator – it's *what* you are communicating that's the problem.

The good news is that it's easier than you think to change negative self-communication. When you change what you communicate in the way that I'm going to show you, you *automatically* change to positive self-communication. In fact, it's so easy that it's a little scary – this book could actually be a one-page leaflet! But if I told you it all right now, you might question it because of its simplicity. You've been putting so much energy and effort into doing the *opposite* that it's going to be much more fun for you to read the book and begin to find it for yourself.

I wonder how far into the book you will be before you 'get it'? When you *do* reach that point, whether it's in the first chapter or the last, every word, sentence or paragraph after it will enhance everything you can learn. You'll be amazed at the simplicity of it all, and wonder why other people can't see it too.

There are exercises for you to complete throughout the book. You can either write your responses straight on to the page, or keep a journal of your progress. It's important that you complete these exercises, because research has proven time and again that people who write down their experiences are more likely to learn from them.

The Canadian psychologist Paul Bloom says that 'The mind is a product of the brain. The mind is what the brain does.' So, what is *your* brain doing? And would you like to *change* it?

As you progress through the programme, you'll start to notice how you can change your mind – psychologically and emotionally in the way that you think – and at the same time, *physically* change the way you look and feel. Try to identify which techniques in particular are working well for you; notice what your lightbulb moments are, and when they occur (as they certainly will!) In doing so, you'll learn how to adapt and change even faster; this is all part of you creating your *own* strategy.

Introducing Mabel

Hi, I'm Mabel,

I've completed this programme, and while I was doing it, I kept a journal of my experiences. I'll be happy to share this with you, but not just yet! First, here's a little bit about me. I was fat (my friends called it 'overweight', but I knew they really meant 'fat') and I didn't like it. In fact, I hated it. I tried many times to lose the fat. Once, when faced with a short-notice invitation to the wedding of a friend I hadn't seen in years, I lived on cabbage soup and boiled eggs for three weeks (yuk!). I certainly <u>looked</u> slimmer, but I spent most of the wedding clenching my buttocks in an effort not to fart. (Honestly, I'm sure I could've let out the tune to the whole Wedding March in perfect time if I'd put my mind to it!)

After that, I tried the high-protein diet (not so fondly remembered as the 'smelly breath' diet by my mates), until even I couldn't bear the smell. I got fed up with people asking me to 'breathe somewhere else', and I also had a constant backache (I learnt why that was when I read this book). Then came membership of a slimming club, where I diligently followed the strict regime, striving to reach what I had been told was my 'ideal weight'. That went quite well for a few weeks, but then I got fed up with measuring and counting <u>everything</u> I ate and started to deviate. For 24 hours prior to the dreaded weekly weigh-in, I would stop eating, surviving on diet cola to stave off hunger pangs. Afterwards, I'd go home via the chip shop and vow to 'start again tomorrow'.

Of course, I've also tried numerous 'celebrity' diets, only to realize that most of these require a very deep purse, a personal chef, or a lot of time available to spend shopping and in the kitchen. I finally decided that I didn't want someone to look at my poo, or scold me publicly when I screwed up – I just wanted to know how to change my shape without denying myself all the foods I love. I wanted to stop craving the foods that made me fat; stop stuffing my face then regretting it later and feeling lousy; and stop settling for poor health. I was fed up with feeling exhausted. I was fed up with feeling fed up! I wanted to be able to get into the nice clothes that had been hanging unworn in my wardrobe for longer than I cared to admit. I knew my overeating was ridiculous, and I was certain that inside me there <u>really was</u> a thin person just waiting to get out – despite the fact that I was sabotaging all my weight-loss efforts and keeping her hidden!

Finally, it dawned on me that I needed to control what went on in my <u>head</u> before I could control what went into my mouth. That was a revelation! Actually, I can't believe it took me so long to work it out! When I started this programme I was a bit sceptical, and while I was doing it, it wasn't all plain sailing – I learnt the difference between 'simple' and 'easy' very early on! I want to tell you, though, that I have been where you are now. I'm going to share some of my thoughts and experiences with *you in this book and I hope they inspire you, and maybe even make you smile! Everything you read is real.*

Doing this programme has not only changed my body – it has changed my life. Actually, let me rephrase that: the programme itself didn't change things, I changed my life. I took responsibility for the changes and made them happen in a way that was right for me. You can do this too. You are going to experience a sense of change and achievement that will make you tingle when it becomes a reality! And your story might inspire someone else, as I hope mine inspires you. The only thing that comes close to equalling the incredible feeling of achievement I have now is the hope that I can help others experience it too.

Mabel x

~~~~~~~~~~~~~~~~~~~~~~~

Measuring Up

Before you begin, take some measurements so you can accurately monitor your progress at certain stages of the programme. First, weigh yourself on some reliable scales. These must be the *only* scales you use in the following months, because scales vary according to how they are calibrated and where you position them, and your weight varies depending what time of day you weigh yourself, so all these things need to be constant and repeatable.

Next, get a tape measure and measure the sites shown on the table below (if possible, get someone to do it for you). Record the measurements in the table below, or in your journal.

Date	Weight	Arm 1	Arm 2	Bust	Tummy	Hips	Thigh 1	Thigh 2

If you would like to use a fuller weight chart, you can download one for free from my website, www.powertochange.me.uk. Click on the *Think More, Eat Less* link on the home page and type in the password 'Positive Attitude'.

When you measure yourself, make sure the tape is level and not twisted. And *always measure at the widest point for each body site*: there's no point measuring your waist if below it you have a bulging tummy – that's why the table says 'tummy' and not waist! For some people, the widest point for the tummy measurement will be on their belly button; for others (depending on where they store their fat), it may be several centimetres below. It's the same thing with your hips – technically, you would take the measurement in line with the end of the pubic bone, but adapt this if this is not your *widest point*. When you measure individual thighs, do exactly the same thing.

You can't beat noticing that your clothes are getting looser, so, in addition to measuring yourself, find a pair of jeans or trousers and a top that are currently too tight for you and try them on every week so that you can see a real difference. Remember, scales can be unreliable and your body weight can fluctuate by 1.8 kg (4 lbs) within any given day, so you *must* use other measures of your progress to get a balanced view of your progress.

I recommend that you *do not repeat any of the measurements*, including your weight, until you have completed the two-week Healthy Starter Plan in chapter 12. After that, measure yourself once a week, and weigh yourself once every two weeks at the most. *You don't need to weigh yourself every day* – this is not a diet, it is a plan for your mind and body that will get you to a healthy place physically that just happens to include being a healthy weight. How you approach the programme mentally is vital to your success. If possible, get together with a friend or a small group of friends at a set time each week to take the measurements. Research has shown that the support of a group can be very beneficial. I must add though, this is *only* the case if the overall mental attitude is one of support and encouragement. It is not a chance to get together for a right old moan, or to put the world to rights! Be disciplined and use the group only for encouragement and support, and for sharing ideas. You can also join our Facebook group, *Think More Eat Less* for support and on-going tips and updates – you can also ask me questions.

Chapter 1

'I GOTTA FEELING'

Why are you reading this book? Just take a moment to consider that question properly. If your answer is something like, 'Because I am fed up with being fat and I want to be slim', how do you know that's what you want? Seriously, how do you *know*?

Consider this concept – you don't 'have' feelings, you 'do' feelings. Take love, for example. Think of a person, or a pet, or even a thing that you love deeply. Would you say, 'I *have* love for them', or would you say, 'I love them', making love something you *experience* or *do* rather than *have*. Forget the rules of English grammar for a moment, and think of feelings as verbs, in that you *do* them as opposed to *have* them. Now think about how you are 'doing' knowing that you want to be slim. At some level, that 'knowing' is based on a feeling.

This book is going to teach you so many exciting things about how you 'do' feelings. We are taught that we process all the information we receive through our senses in our brains, and of course, technically, that's

1

true. However, there is a clear mind–body connection that ensures we transmute (change and adapt) those chemical brain processes into sensations and feelings in different parts of our bodies. For example, have you ever felt weak at the knees? You don't have a brain in your knees, so how is it that you can feel something there that is based on an *emotion*? We know we have nerves in our knees and that they tell the brain when our knees are hurt, that makes perfect sense, but how can an emotion create a feeling in our knees that literally makes them weaken or wobble? There are other emotion-based sensations that present themselves as physical symptoms, including butterflies in the tummy or tension headaches.

Your Mind Affects Your Body

The reality is this: there is on-going, non-stop communication between your mind and your body. You are *one* unit made up of *two* different corresponding parts. And here comes a really important point: one of those parts is much more powerful than the other. Your *mind* can directly affect the health of your body. Your mind also drives your behaviours and your body is simply a visible representation of what has been going on in your mind – all your thoughts about yourself. Put simply, you (and everyone else) can see the effects of what goes on in your mind by looking at the state and shape of your body. If you constantly think, 'I can't be bothered', you are likely to have a different body shape from someone who thinks, 'I *will* make the effort'.

In modern medicine, the body has long been treated as a totally separate entity from the mind, often at great cost to the patient. Louise Hay, the founder of Hay House (who publish this book), was one of the very first people to recognize that our thoughts and our feelings affect our health in very specific ways – either positively or negatively – and that we can use our minds to change the health of our bodies. Today, many others are following in her wake, developing new ways of thinking and behaving that can positively impact on our health – physically, mentally and emotionally. Recently, the ground-breaking American scientist Bruce Lipton wrote *The Biology of Belief*, an astonishing account of how our thoughts *literally* change the biology of our cells. The idea that our minds affect our bodies had been dismissed as 'New Age' thinking for years, but it can now be proven at the chemical level, right down to changes in DNA. I will teach you much more about this later in the book.

Turning Information Into Action

Let's look at how your emotions drive your behaviour. If you have two opposing feelings, the strongest of these will determine how you behave. It's not possible to feel good and bad at the same time, because one feeling will dominate. For example, you want to be slimmer than you are now, yet a part of your mind still wants the feeling it gets when you eat too much. Up until now, that has been the dominant feeling and that's why you are overweight. So, do you want to change that feeling now?

Exercise
· · · · · · · · ·

Stand in front of a full-length mirror with as few clothes on as possible. Spend a few minutes (or as long as it takes) having a good look at yourself as a physical being. Allow yourself to acknowledge all the things you don't like about being fat. You may think, 'I just hate it!' but try to consider exactly *what* it is that you hate. For example, you might think: 'I hate getting undressed in front of someone', or 'I get out of breath whenever I go upstairs', or 'I can't buy the clothes I want'. You get the kind of thing? Now make a list of the top six things you hate about being fat and write them in the table below or in your journal; leave the second column blank for the next part of the exercise. Make sure you start each point with, 'I hate'.

WHAT I HATE ABOUT BEING FAT	HOW THIS MAKES ME FEEL
1.	1.
2.	2.
3.	3.
4.	4.
5.	5.
6.	6.

Now think about how each of these things makes you *feel*. For example, 'Getting undressed in front of someone makes me feel ashamed and embarrassed', or 'Getting out of breath makes me feel unhealthy', or 'Not being able to buy the clothes I want makes me feel frumpy'. When you have identified the *feelings* you associate with each of the six things you hate about being fat, write them down in the second column. Make sure you start each one with, 'I feel'.

Why do you think that, despite hating these feelings, you have still been *doing* the behaviours that make you fat?

The next step is to identify six things that you've been doing on a regular, even daily, basis that have been making you fat, and keeping you fat. Your answers might be: 'I eat chocolate and sweets every day', or 'I keep eating even when I've had enough', or 'I buy and eat junk food', or 'I dish up more than I need', or 'I sit down too much instead of being active – I'm lazy', or 'I eat fast without thinking about what or how much I'm eating'. Spend some time now and honestly identify what your *behaviours* are. Write them down in the table below, making sure you start each one with 'I' so you can begin to take responsibility and associate deeply with what you are learning. Remember, this is all about *you*! Leave the second column blank for the next part of the exercise.

BEHAVIOURS	DESIRED FEELING
1.	1.
2.	2.
3.	3.
4.	4.
5.	5.
6.	6.

Now think about the *feeling* you get when you are 'doing' these behaviours, or more importantly, the feeling you *want* to get! For example, you might say: 'I want to feel comforted', or 'I want to feel full and satisfied', or 'I want to feel as though I don't care about being fat'. Write your answers in the second column. If you can't think of a feeling – think again! All behaviours, big or small, generate a feeling of some kind, and doing nothing is by default doing something. Often, especially with comfort eating, the desired feeling is to feel numbness – to blank out the negative thoughts you are currently experiencing. Whatever the feeling is, it ends with 'and happy', otherwise you wouldn't want to feel it. Even if you do something that makes you feel *unhappy*, there's some benefit in your feeling unhappy and that makes it a worthwhile feeling.

Do You Want To Harm Or To Heal?

Have you ever stopped to ask yourself how you actually benefit from this kind of eating behaviour? Would you suddenly get a knife and slash away at your arm to relieve boredom, or to feel comforted? Of course not – that would be madness! There's a name for that type of behaviour – self-harming – and it's a symptom of great mental distress. Well, I have news for you: overeating and making your body fat is a clear case of self-harming! In fact, in some ways, it's even worse than the more obvious forms because it's insidious. That means it's sneaky and deceptive – it's self-harming by stealth. It's so stealthy that you can convince yourself you are not self-harming – but you are. Let me say that again, in another way:

Every time you overeat or drink high-calorie junk, especially when you don't need food for energy (i.e.

when you are already satisfied), you are deliberately harming yourself.

Overeating is no better than self-harming with a knife – you just kid yourself that it is. When you harm with a knife there is clear evidence of the harm in the form of scars. But look again, your excess body fat is clearer and more visible than any scar – it's a sign to you and everyone else that you have been self-harming.

It's time for some honesty now. When you eat to numb emotional pain, or because you don't think you are worth the effort it takes to be healthy, you are using the same technique that an alcoholic or a drug addict uses to bury, numb or forget an unpleasant feeling or difficult circumstances. Rather than changing their circumstances, they artificially and temporarily change how they *feel*. The trouble is, when they regain normal consciousness they crave a return to the escapism of drink or drugs. Instead of dealing with their problems, they amplify and add to them. Being a 'foodoholic' might not sound as bad as being an alcoholic, but believe me when I say it is – if not worse. Shocked? If so, good! It's time for a wake-up call. Remember this:

Overeating is not a form of escapism – it's self-harming.

Some people are 'professional victims' of life's problems, deriving pleasure from feeling unlucky and unhappy because it defines them. Does being fat define you? Is it *who* you are, or is it *what* you are? Think about this question and write your answer down below:

Being fat is _____

If you think it's *who* you are, then you are wrong. Being fat is not who you are, it's merely *what* you are, and you can start to change that right now. Being fat is a physical symptom, or indicator, of your behaviours, in the same way that a scar is the symptom of a past trip or fall. But while some scars are for life, being fat does not have to be for life. It does not define you unless you choose to let it, and opt for becoming a victim. I doubt that this is the case with you, though, because you are reading this book. That tells me (and you) that you want to change and that you want to know how to do it.

Exercise

Now I want you to think of ways of generating the feelings you want through behaviours that are *not* self-harming and fat-making. This exercise is something you can return to again and again, as certain things can make you happy on one day, but not on another. For example, if the feeling you want is 'to escape', or to 'feel numb' in order to avoid a negative thought, watching a movie or a natural history programme like *Planet Earth* will completely take your focus away from you and on to the bigger picture, which is a good thing. However, if it's a gorgeous sunny day, shutting yourself indoors to watch TV may not be the best idea. Similarly, if you want to feel happy and you love walking, taking a hike may have the desired effect in fine weather, but if you make yourself do it when it's cold and wet, you may end up with a different feeling than the one you want!

As you think about this, try to come up with a variety of ways of generating the feelings you desire. I've given some examples below; write your ideas in the blank columns.

DESIRED FEELING	ALTERNATIVE BEHAVIOURS
To escape	Have a long soak in the bath with an inspiring book
To be in control	Make or create something – write a poem, paint a picture, make a meal from a recipe
To be happy	Listen to music; look at photographs of happy occasions; call or visit friends
To spoil myself	Have a pampering beauty treatment; go somewhere special (not food related)

Now, it may seem like I'm pointing out the obvious here, but there's a good reason for this, so bear with me. You need to start believing and accepting that if you want to look and *be* different physically, you have to *do* different things. This becomes easier if you take some time to think about what you can do *instead* of overeating that will still give you the feelings you want.

The problem with the whole concept of dieting is that people do things that they don't enjoy in order to reach a goal. Then, when they get there (assuming they can do what they don't enjoy for long enough), they naturally stop doing the things they didn't enjoy and the weight goes back on. This is because all the reasons they overate in the first place are still there and they haven't come up with an alternative behaviour to meet those needs! But *you* are not going to make that mistake – you are going to address this issue of changing your body by changing your mind – for good – are you not?

Exercise

Before we go any further, let me ask you just what it is that you want to achieve with this programme? I mean specifically, which dress size do you want to be? Or for men, which trouser size? Write your answer below:

CURRENT DRESS SIZE	DESIRED DRESS SIZE

I have deliberately not put weight as a goal here, and I will explain why later on in the book, although we *will* take weight into account. We will also add a time frame to this, but for now, focus clearly on what you want to achieve and start to believe it will happen. Start to see in your mind (or visualize) how you will look and feel a month *after* you have achieved your goal, once you are enjoying all the benefits. Then visualize yourself three months after that, then six months, so it is not the actual achieving of the goal that is first and foremost in your mind, but the months *after* you have already achieved it. As you visualize, make sure you take notice of your new behaviours. What do you see yourself doing now you have made the changes and lost the weight? How is it different from how you behaved before?

There are two important times for controlling your thoughts and feelings, and they are influenced by how your brain works, and on what 'wavelength'.

1. **Just before you go to sleep.** When you are relaxed, your brain uses alpha waves and as a result, you are more creative and better able to use your imagination. You will see in a later chapter how vital your imagination is in the process of change, but briefly, if you can see yourself doing something in your mind in a powerful way, then you can also do it 'in reality'. If you visualize in this way often enough, what you are seeing in your mind actually *becomes* your behaviour. Some people do this all the time with negative thoughts and projections. How many times have you heard someone say, 'I *knew* that would

happen!' when things go wrong? They manifested the event through negative visualization – they focused on the worst thing that could happen, literally made a movie out of it in their minds, and it happened! The technique of visualization must only be used with *positive* visualizations, and as you do this repetitively and with purpose, watch how you can change your 'luck' from bad to good.

2. **When you wake up.** From today onward, dedicate at least one minute to seeing yourself as successful in your goal as soon as you wake up and before you go to sleep. Remember to visualize yourself *after* you have achieved your goal. Are you worth two minutes of your time every single day? You'd better believe that you are!

Mabel's Journal

OK, today's the day I start yet another diet! Actually, the Introduction tells me it's not a diet, which is a relief, because I've done enough of those to last a lifetime! Not sure what to expect – this one seems like a very different approach. If it does what it says on the cover, though, I'll be a happy (and slim) girl. In the Introduction it says, 'The mind is what the brain does.' I'm not sure what my brain is doing most of the time, so this should be interesting. I might get more than I bargained for!!

I'm told it's a good idea to keep a journal of my progress as I work through each chapter of the programme, so here goes. Just done the measuring and weighing. This is the heaviest I've ever been! I can't believe it! And I'm a dress size 20. Can I really get down to a size 12?

'I Gotta Feeling' – strange to have a Black Eyed Peas song title as a chapter heading. Already though, I can hear the song playing in my head. I wonder if that's the idea? Is tonight gonna be a good night??

~~~~~~~~~~~~~~~~

Since I finished this chapter, I've been reflecting on the idea that I'm never not communicating... with myself! Seems so obvious now I think about it, but I really do communicate better with just about anyone than I do with myself. Makes me realize that if I spoke to other people the way I 'talk' to myself, I wouldn't have any friends, or a job! Also realized that I struggle with opposing thoughts: on the one hand I want to be slim, on the other, I want to eat and eat! So if the thought that evokes the strongest emotion 'wins', then it's no wonder I'm fat – I'm REALLY emotional about food! And I can't really imagine myself as being slim. I can't really imagine myself winning the lottery either, although I would like to!

Did the mirror exercise today – that was painful! Had to use the mirror in the spare room because I won't have a full-length one in my bedroom. Interesting that on my list of 'Things I hate about being fat', number one was, 'Looking in the mirror and seeing myself!' All I could come up with when asked, 'How does this make you feel?' was 'Like shit!'. This might not be as easy as I thought. Even though I know exactly what has made me fat – eating rubbish and sitting on my butt too much – I have never really thought about eating to get a _feeling_. Sometimes I eat just to relieve boredom, but other times it really is to push a negative thought or experience out of my head by focusing on food instead.

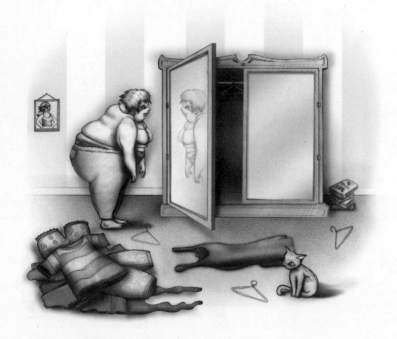

OMG! I've just read the bit about overeating being just like self-harming!!!! There was a girl at college who always wore long sleeves, even in hot weather, to cover up the scars on her arms from self-harming. Everyone felt so bad for her but they didn't know what to do or say to help her. I wonder if people feel sorry for me for harming myself with food??!!! I don't like that thought one bit. Definitely going to work on my 'Things to do instead of eating to get a good feeling' list. I'm going to start now by having a soak in the bath instead of rushing in the shower for two minutes.

~~~~~~~~~~~~~~~~~~~~~~

Since reading this chapter I've spent the last three nights visualizing myself as slim. Not easy – I can sort of see it, but not very clearly, and it doesn't really look like me. I bought a magazine today with a not-too-skinny model on the cover, and pasted a photo of my head on her body – that helped. Going to look at her every day and focus on my end goal. Wow, this book has certainly got my brain cells going! I am cautiously optimistic now that I actually can change :o)

Chapter 2

THOUGHTS ARE 'THINGS'

You are a spiritual being. I'm not talking about religion – your beliefs on that are not relevant to this concept. What I mean is that the air around you – the atmosphere or the 'ether' – is not just empty space, it is full of 'information'. And your thoughts are also information – they are real 'things'. Although you can't see them, they have a substance that gives them an energetic force. This concept has become much more widely known in recent years, as films and books like *The Secret* have encouraged people to use their unconscious minds to focus on drawing to them what they desire. This principle is popular, but in reality, in order to draw something to you, you also have to practically *do* whatever it takes to make that happen. You will learn how to do just that in this book. You will learn how to combine your mental attitude and focus to drive your unconscious mind to create the behaviours that will bring you what you want – a slimmer, healthier body – along with practical techniques for your conscious mind to engage in that will help make it happen.

This kind of thinking is not new, though. In fact, it first appeared in the brilliant works of the American author Napoleon Hill, who wrote, among other things, the hugely successful book *Think and Grow Rich* (1937). This great book's title belies the fact that it is essentially about how to *think differently* in order to achieve any physical goal – not just a financial one. Napoleon Hill's works have influenced most, if not all, of today's self-help gurus, and the origins of Neuro-Linguistic Programming, or NLP, can be found in much of his work, in particular the concept of 'modelling', which we will explore later in the book.

The First Ever Self-Help Guru

In 1908, Hill, then a young journalist, interviewed the powerful industrialist Andrew Carnegie for an article he was writing. Originally from Scotland, Carnegie had emigrated with his family to America at the age of 13. He worked in a factory and in other lowly positions before going on to found a steel company that was valued at $480 million when he retired in 1901. He then started to give his fortune away to good causes – his strongly held belief was that the rich are merely 'trustees' of their wealth and are under a moral obligation to distribute it in ways that promote the welfare and happiness of the common man. He also believed that anyone could achieve the enormous success that he, and others like him, had enjoyed.

Carnegie took a liking to Hill, and commissioned him to undertake the task of analyzing and then sharing the methods he had used so effectively in his business.

Hill then spent the next 20 years interviewing some of the most successful people in the USA at the time – including Thomas Edison, F. W. Woolworth and Henry Ford – drawing out and then 'modelling' their thought processes. The sum total of that study appears in *Think and Grow Rich*. Hill set down 13 key principles, and I will be covering these in this programme. I've listed them all for you below, because they can be adapted, and are fully relevant to achieving a *physical* goal as well as a *monetary* one.

The 13 principles of Napoleon Hill:

1. **Desire** – You must create an overwhelming desire to achieve your specific goal.

2. **Faith** – You must have absolute faith in your ability to achieve your goal.

3. **Autosuggestion** – You must learn to accept your own positive suggestions.

4. **Specialized knowledge** – You must do whatever it takes to learn any method or technique you need in order to achieve your goal.

5. **Imagination** – Through the power of your imagination, you can create real scenarios and create change.

6. **Organized planning** – You must have a specific strategy.

7. **Decision** – You must make a definite decision and master the act of procrastination.

8.   **Persistence** – You must develop the ability to continue toward your goal whatever distractions, or temporary lack of success, occur along the way. This is the power of will.

9.   **The Master Mind principle** – This is the driving force of combined thoughts for a common goal.

10. **Transmutation** – To change one form of energy into another.

11. **Subconscious** – The connecting link between our senses and our recording process.

12. **The Brain** – A broadcasting and receiving station for thoughts.

13. **Sixth Sense** – The means through which 'Infinite Intelligence' (more about this later) can communicate and respond to any individual effort.

Thinking Outside the Box

We will explore these principles in more detail as we go on. You will learn how to adapt and apply many of them to *you*, and your desired goal of weight loss. These are well-established, tried and tested techniques that have been used by some of the most successful people in the world to help them achieve their goals – most of which were considerably harder than learning how to eat a bit less and move a bit more!

   One of the key findings of Napoleon Hill's research was the 'power of thought'. We will be looking at this concept on many levels throughout the book, as conscious thinking, unconscious thinking, and the power of thought as a tool for communication through the 'ether'. So, it's time to set aside your traditional ways of thinking and try something new. Be curious! What do you think is the best thing that could happen?

Your thoughts truly are 'things' and just because you can't see them, it doesn't mean they are not there. After all, if you drop something, you know the power of gravity will cause it to fall to the floor. You don't question it. You can't see the gravity, but you can see the effect it has. Your thoughts are just the same – you can't see them, but you can see their *effects*. You just haven't linked the two together yet – so let's try that now.

Where Your Thoughts And Behaviours Come From

Are you aware that you have two minds? You have a conscious mind and an unconscious (or subconscious) mind. In your conscious mind, you can process approximately seven pieces of information at any one time (plus or minus two). Every other thought you have is in your unconscious mind. Now just think about that for a moment, because a thought can also be described as a 'message' or a 'signal', and your body is a mass of signals constantly passing between your cells and your brain.

Right now, there are trillions of messages whizzing around your body at a very high rate of vibration. They are telling your body when to breathe and how much CO_2 to expel; they are monitoring your blood pressure, monitoring how much blood goes through your kidneys, which cells need repairing or renewing… you get the idea? If you were aware of all these messages, you'd be completely overwhelmed with information, so there is an ingenious, and essential, division between your conscious mind and your unconscious mind.

The illustration below explains, very simply, how the conscious and unconscious minds work. It shows an iceberg: a huge, mountain-like structure with its top *above* the water line and the bulk of it, the bit that determines its strength, *below* the water line. The conscious mind is shown as the top of the iceberg, the tiny bit above the water line; and your unconscious mind – the really important bit – is the major part below the water line.

Your Two Minds

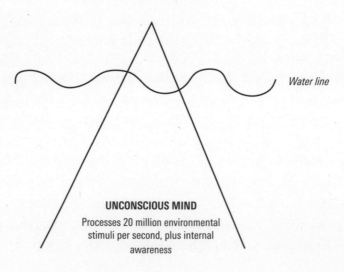

CONSCIOUS MIND
Processes 7 pieces of information (+/- 2)

Water line

UNCONSCIOUS MIND
Processes 20 million environmental
stimuli per second, plus internal
awareness

In the first chapter, we looked at 'how' you think and feel. This is done by your 'conscious mind' – the bit above the water line, where you process your environment. For example, as you read this, how comfortable are you? What are your surroundings like? As you focus on the words you are reading now, are you saying them out loud in your head? Are you adding your own comments to specific points? All of these things are in your conscious mind. Below the water line, in your unconscious mind, is a database of everything that has ever happened to you. Some of this information will never reach your conscious mind, but it can still have a huge impact on your thoughts, and therefore on your behaviours. It could be experiences from childhood that you have long forgotten *consciously*, but these have formed your belief system into what it is today, determining how you think and behave.

The 'water line' acts as a filter system that determines exactly what information makes it through to your unconscious mind. When you have an experience, you instantly decide whether the information is worth keeping, and so file it in your unconscious mind, or delete it – millions of minor signals and messages are filtered out in this way. Other experiences, or pieces of information, do get through the filtration process, but only because we adapt or distort them to make them 'fit' a particular belief system.

Creating 'Associations'

By manipulating information in this way, we can sometimes record information incorrectly. A good example of this is when smokers convince themselves that smoking will not cause terrible suffering and disease, and a painful death, even though they 'know' consciously that it will. They delete crucial evidence and then distort what's left, creating different associations to make it acceptable. For example, when young people start smoking they tell themselves, 'It makes me look cool in front of my mates'. This creates a positive association with smoking and the unconscious mind accepts this distortion as true and installs the behaviour. As they get older and wiser, those people learn this is not true consciously, but the unconscious pattern has been set and until that association is broken, the unconscious belief and the behaviour of smoking persists, despite conscious protests.

All it took to install the negative behaviour was a *powerful thought combined with a strong emotion*. A thought *without* emotion cannot be converted into a belief or a behaviour – you must have the emotional intensity of *feeling* to connect with the thought – to give it the power to create the behaviour. In the same way, to delete a behaviour, you must combine an *opposing* thought with a powerful emotion to delete the connection. For example, have you ever eaten something that made you so ill that you still couldn't touch it, months or even years later? Last year I got food poisoning from a lamb tagine, and every time I see it on a menu now I shudder, and wouldn't consider ordering it. It's all about association.

Here's a simple way of looking at it:

Thought + intense emotion = association = behaviours created

or

Thought + intense emotion = association = behaviours destroyed

Below is another 'iceberg' illustration. This one explains how the conscious mind feeds the unconscious mind information in the form of conscious 'thoughts' – passing them through the 'water line' based on the intensity of the emotion, and the associations we subsequently attach to it.

The conscious mind (via the senses and general processing of information) 'sends' information deep into the unconscious mind to be cross-referenced, matched and filed in the correct place – i.e. in line with our established beliefs and values. The unconscious mind then collates all this information and, based on what has been received, 'sends' its instructions back to the conscious mind to create and drive everyday behaviours.

You can think of the conscious mind as representing workers reporting into head office (the unconscious mind), which creates policies based on how that information compares with its existing database and then sends back strong signals for how to behave.

Where Our Behaviours Come From

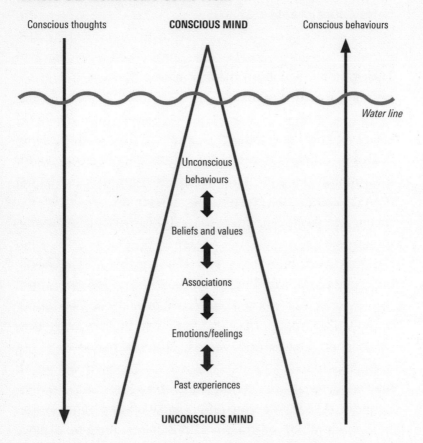

How Your Thinking Drives Your Behaviour

Later in the book, you'll find an exercise that will enable you to make use of this process to great effect, but in the meantime, here's a way of looking at it in very simple terms. When you were young, your mother told you not to touch the oven because it's hot. Now either you believed her, or you actually touched the oven yourself and learnt that if you touch this thing it hurts. Information was combined with emotion and association to create a behaviour – in this case, the behaviour was to keep away from the oven!

This is how you learn everything you now know – by association. Put another way, if you decide something is important then it influences you; if it's not important, it doesn't. That's why when someone you know, or even worse, love, insults you, it hurts more than if the insult came from someone you have a low opinion of, or don't know. What creates the all-important association? You know the answer of course – it's a thought.

When you are thinking about whether or not to associate pleasure or pain with something, your mind processes the associations it has already made. For instance, if someone says to you, 'Let's go to London for the weekend', and you have been to London before, your mind will use that as a reference. If you had a good time on the previous occasion you will respond positively, and if you had a bad time, you will respond negatively. If you have never been to London, your mind will search for similar experiences and will project what you think will happen over the weekend to make its decision. Simply put: your mind likes patterns – it likes things that are the same. If a particular situation has evoked a particular thought, emotion or behaviour in the past, your mind is likely to stick to that pattern, unless you change your thinking and make new associations.

This is why so many people stay in abusive relationships – although they hate their situation, they are afraid of being alone, or worried about where they will go if they leave. If they stay with what they know, at least they know what they are dealing with. Have you heard the saying, 'better the devil you know'? Well, that belief is responsible for a lot of people not changing, or not trying something new. We like to stay within our comfort zones; our unconscious mind likes and desires a sense of security and it gets that from doing what it knows. Until you change that thinking, and start to think that things will be better another way, you will be stuck in the rut.

SHIT – How Much Do You Have?

It has been said that of the thousands of thoughts we have every day, over 80 per cent are the same negative ones repeated over and over again. So, it's time for some new thinking! You are just one thought away from changing everything. Are you ready for that? Every thought is a piece of the jigsaw puzzle that makes up who you are.

I have been working with people who want to change how they think and feel (as well as how they look) for more than 20 years, and it's my belief that many of the negative thoughts those people had weren't even their own – by that I mean that they accepted the negative imprint from someone else. In other words, they accepted other people's thinking as their own. My advice to you is to *stop* letting other people's **S**ystemic **H**armful **I**nvasive **T**houghts (SHIT) affect you!

Systemic – it goes all the way through you
Harmful – it hurts
Invasive – it gets below the skin
Thoughts – define you

It's their SHIT, not yours. You can create a much better thought process of your own. So the next time you find yourself thinking something negative, just remember: that thought is SHIT. Choose a better one. Your internal voice is a representation of your thoughts and as such, it can be controlled and changed. Most people leave their internal voice on the default setting, though. They play what they are used to hearing – what they know. They don't make the effort to tune into a different voice, just like you would re-tune a radio and see what else is on if you didn't like what you were listening to.

If you really *must* accept other people's thoughts, then surround yourself with positive, optimistic people who really achieve what they want. I'm not talking about money, although that often comes to positive thinkers, but in all areas – physically, mentally, spiritually and emotionally. Be around people who possess the qualities that you would like to have. Listen to what they say, talk to them in a bit more detail about how they think, pay attention to their actions and notice how many more positive outcomes they have than 'unlucky' people. Of course, this doesn't mean that every single thought brings a positive outcome. Or does it? There's a nice thought!

You Become What You Think You Will Become

Your thoughts define you. You must have had the thought, 'I want to be slimmer', or you wouldn't be reading this. But you *are* reading it. I invite you to continue to read... patiently. Stop and pause regularly to reflect on what you are learning. This is not a novel, although it does tell the story of *how you became you*, and what you can become if you really want to. Of course, like all good stories, it leaves you to fill in the really important bits! So, as you read patiently – and possibly more slowly than you would normally read a book, so you can allow your thoughts to form – you might just awaken a genuine interest within your mind in how to change. As you take the simple steps and complete the exercises, know also that *how you think as you read will determine your success with this programme.* If you think about it, this could be the very last time you ever have to consciously make the effort to get the body you want. That could be both an incentive and a relief, depending on how you think about it!

Can you remember how exciting learning something new was when you were young? To a child, even learning to walk is exciting. As children we don't process the thought, 'I keep falling over – I'll never be able to walk, I'm a failure!' We just keep getting up and trying again until we learn from our experience, adjusting our balance until we can not only walk, but run, dance, hop, skip and jump, too! It's no coincidence that when you were a child you learnt at a much faster rate than you do now. No doubt the subject you most liked at school was taught by your favourite teacher; he or she made learning fun and interesting, and inspired you.

Re-create that teacher now as you read through the pages of this book, and let the knowledge and understanding unfold. With every page you turn, open a new page in your mind with pleasure and anticipation; be eager to learn and as eager to please yourself as you might once have been eager to please your favourite teacher! Fifty per cent of everything you need to know about how to change and be the person you want to be, physically and emotionally, is in this book, the other 50 per cent is already within you, perhaps hidden or buried. As you read, your own 50 per cent will be revealed to you through your thoughts. It might come to you piece by piece, or perhaps in one big epiphany moment! I wonder which way you think it will happen? I am curious and excited for you!

Exercise
. . . .

Think about the negative thoughts you've had on a regular basis that allowed you to self-harm by overeating and under-exercising. Are they your own SHIT thoughts? Or are they someone else's SHIT thoughts? Who made you think, and therefore feel, that you weren't worth the effort it takes to have a wonderful, healthy, vibrant body? A friend? A relative? A partner? A teacher? A parent? The media? If the influence didn't come from someone else (and it probably did, even if you don't realize it yet) then what SHIT thoughts did you generate *yourself* that allowed you to abuse and overwrite your instinctive desire for survival and health?

In the table below, write the name of the person who gave you the SHIT thought, what the thought was, and what has been the outcome of keeping that SHIT thought.

31

PERSON	THOUGHT	OUTCOME
Fred	I am not good enough	Eat for comfort = fat
Me	I am stupid	Might as well be fat and stupid = overeat

The original thought was accepted with such emotion (even if it was a negative emotion) that it became a belief that generated its own set of behaviours. You are just one thought away from changing that – or have you already started to think differently? We will look at beliefs in a little more detail later on, for now, focus on changing your thinking and your associations.

From Incompetence To Competence

I told you earlier that your mind likes doing things that are the same. Well, now I'm going to guide you through the process of change. Before you decided that you wanted to change, were you going along thinking there wasn't really a problem with your weight and size? There's a stage *before* the change process and it's called

'Unconscious Incompetence'. This means you are really bad at doing something (in this case looking after your body) but you don't yet realize it. Have you ever worked with someone who is hopeless at their job but who thinks they are great at it? That's Unconscious Incompetence. (You only have to watch TV talent shows to see more examples of Unconscious Incompetence!) While *you* are at this stage, no changes can take place.

Then comes a light bulb moment – perhaps you see an unflattering photograph of yourself and you suddenly realize you are bad at something (in this case looking after yourself), but you don't know how to do things differently. This is called 'Conscious Incompetence' – you are bad at looking after your body, but now at least you know you are bad at it! This is a good stage to be at because it can be a springboard for change, as long as you *want* to change. At this point you need some intervention, some help or information that will tell you how and what to change. *You are reading that help right now!* When you learn new techniques, like the ones in this book, they don't become automatic right away. In fact, your unconscious mind might even resist change and try to draw you back to what you know, especially if it thinks you are going to go on a diet and it has negative associations with past attempts.

So, this means that, at first, you must *consciously* make the changes – you must literally think about doing the new behaviours in place of the old ones. This stage is called 'Conscious Competence', which means you can do it, but only when you *think* about it. This stage feels different; some people say it's uncomfortable, but I think they are confusing uncomfortable with 'different'. It feels different *at first*, but very soon (within a few weeks) you get used to the new behaviours and you don't have to think about them quite as much. They become automatic. When you reach this stage, you will automatically use the new behaviours instead of the old ones, without thinking consciously – this is called 'Unconscious Competence'. You have now re-wired your thinking and changed your default setting.

Here are the stages again:

1. **Unconscious Incompetence** = unaware of behaviours
⬇
2. **Conscious Incompetence** = aware of behaviours
⬇

New Skill, Information or Learning

3. **Conscious Competence** = think to activate the new behaviours
⬇
4. **Unconscious Competence** = automatically do the new behaviours

A good example of this process takes place when we are learning to drive. At first, we have to consciously think about *everything*, the clutch, the gear shift, the accelerator, the visual checks – it's almost overwhelming! But think how quickly after you passed your test you began to drive at the same time as chatting or listening to the radio. You went from consciously generating the thoughts you wanted to doing them automatically, without conscious thinking.

Doing It Without Thinking

What other things are you so good at that you can do them without thinking? How many times do you go and get something to eat 'without thinking', for example? That's Unconscious Incompetence. The new thoughts and behaviours you are generating right now in your conscious thinking will become automatic the more you exercise them. If you only had one driving lesson per month, how long would it have taken you to get to Unconscious Competence, compared to if you'd had two or more lessons per week? In the same way, the more effort you can put in right now to changing the thoughts you are having *consciously*, the quicker you will automatically, and seemingly without effort, start making the choices that will give you the body you want.

Through this process – and being aware that you can choose to change – you truly have *free will*. This means you can stop being the victim of your programming, especially as it's other people's SHIT.

It's not about willpower, it's about will-full thinking! But *you* get to choose your thoughts, so stop listening to the same old SHIT and start thinking *consciously*. Think of this as a course in learning to drive – but one in which you learn to drive your brain rather than a car! Your only limitation is what you *think* you can achieve. As Henry Ford once said: 'Whether a man thinks he can or thinks he can't, he is probably right.'

Just *knowing* something isn't enough to actually *do* it, though. After all, you already have a pretty good idea of what to eat, or what not to eat to lose weight, don't you?

Of course you do. Later in the book, I will introduce you to a really simple way of thinking about foods that will help you to put into practice everything you've learnt. No more 'eating without thinking'. Remember this: 'Knowledge is knowing a tomato is a fruit; Wisdom is not putting it in a fruit salad.' Did you ever look at a tomato and think, 'That would be lovely in a fruit salad!'? Probably not, so the thoughts you apply to what you learn determine your behaviour.

Mabel's Journal

Interesting. I watched The Secret a couple of years ago, but I've never thought about it in relation to weight loss. Intrigued to read more now – this really is a different approach. I Googled Napoleon Hill as well. He was quite a character. It seems he was the first ever celebrity life coach of sorts! There are some very old-fashioned concepts in his 13 steps to success, yet they seem surprisingly relevant given that the book they are in was published in the 1950s. Not sure whether I've got past achieving step two yet, but then that's why I bought this book – I don't know how to yet!

Note to self – work more on building faith in my own ability.

Thinking outside the box reminds me of a test I was once given where I had join the dots without taking the pen off the page and only using four strokes. I couldn't work it out until someone showed me how to 'think outside the box' – then it seemed so easy I couldn't believe I hadn't seen it for myself! I wonder if anyone got the answer without being shown? If so, I'd like to have their brain!

Read the bit about having two minds today – made total sense. The diagram of the iceberg and what information goes in = what behaviours come out was revealing! I can see how much my past has influenced the way I think and feel, and how I've used food as a comfort when it is actually harming me. I've never really understood how people can carry on doing something that is so harmful. I gave up smoking after I lost a close relative to lung cancer; there's no way I'm going to increase my chances of having that! Yet I have been doing the same thing with overeating and stupidly been unable to stop myself.

This summer, the singer Amy Winehouse died. The saddest thing of all was not the loss of her as a person or her talent, although of course that was incredibly sad, but just the inevitability of it. Everyone but her could see it coming. I guess she always thought there was plenty of time to change, but then she ran out of time. Am I doing the same thing to myself with food?

OMG! I've just read the bit about SHIT thoughts!!! Soooo true. Have been thinking about where my SHIT thoughts have actually come from, and more importantly, how I can get rid of them, especially as most of them aren't even mine! Here are the first ones to go:

I am fat. I am ugly. I am stupid.

I feel better after writing them down! Now I can see them in black and white, I can't believe I said those things to myself. Definitely SHIT thoughts... Just screwed up the bit of paper and put it in the bin. That felt good! I, Mabel, am changing!! I am getting rid of everyone else's SHIT thoughts. I'm definitely feeling the tide turning in my thinking and getting quite cross with myself for not seeing it before. Still, better late than never, and I'm actually feeling very motivated! Getting a sense of strength and determination I haven't had for as long as I can remember. Feels good :o)

~~~~~~~~~~~

Went out with some of my mates last night. Most of them spent the whole time eating chips and other rubbish and moaning about their weight. What were they thinking!!!? For the first time, I wasn't one of them. I totally shocked everyone by ordering tuna steak and salad with new potatoes (it was surprisingly nice!). Felt very proud. I know it's only one meal, but I really feel like I'm starting to change.

While I was driving to work today I thought about 'how' I was driving without actually thinking about it! I found it really difficult to go back to feeling the clutch, checking the mirrors etc. in a conscious way. I just do it! Can I really get to that stage with eating good food – automatically, without even thinking?? Went to the supermarket at lunchtime and imagined I was having a shopping lesson. I paid close attention to everything on display and actually thought about what I was buying. It was surprising how many things I picked up out of habit – without thinking. I can obviously eat unhealthily in an Unconsciously Incompetent way, so I must be able to turn that around and eat well in an Unconsciously Competent way!!

Chapter 3

THE CHEMISTRY OF A THOUGHT

So, now you know you are only ever a thought away from getting what you want. You know that a thought is a 'thing', and that it has an energy and a force – just like gravity – even though you can't see it. Now for the really cool bit – when you project your thoughts out into the 'ether' (the word for the universal space around us) as powerful visualizations, images and words, then you can begin to make changes you never dreamt were possible. You will find opportunities opening up for you as you begin to attract a more positive influence in your life.

Your Thoughts Are Energetic Signals

When the Italian inventor Guglielmo Marconi told his friends he had discovered a way to transmit sounds through the ether without wires, they had him arrested and taken to a mental asylum for examination! Yet in 1909 Marconi shared the Nobel Prize in Physics with Karl Ferdinand Braun 'in recognition of their contributions to the development of wireless telegraphy'. Radio waves were initially called 'etheric' waves, because they pass through the ether. And because thought waves are not dissimilar to radio waves, it follows that our thoughts contain information that has been up-scaled; information that can be communicated at a level beyond human speech or vision.

Wherever you are, have a look around right now. What do you see? Furniture, people, trees? But what's in the space in between those things; in the space you can't see? Have you ever thought of this space – or 'ether' – as a conductor of information? Sounds a little crazy? Think again. When did you last make a call on a mobile phone? How do you think the sound of your voice reached the person you were talking to? Did you see the words leave your phone and fly through the air? Of course not – but they did!

How does this happen? Well, everything in life vibrates (or resonates) at a certain frequency, and the ether responds to these varying levels of vibration and exchanges information. In a phone call, it exchanges the information of the sound of your voice between the phones. This is possible because in the Scottish scientist Alexander Graham Bell, the inventor of the telephone in the 1870s and an expert on vibration, believed that it was possible to send messages or 'information' through the ether. Today, thanks to his work and his understanding of 'vibrational energy', when you make a phone call the sound of your voice is 'scaled down', or transformed into a vibration that can be sent through the ether, picked up by a receiving station, and 'up-scaled' to become audible words and sounds once more. Pretty cool, huh?

If your thoughts are signals that are transported through the ether, then, I have two questions for you:

1. **What thoughts are you putting out there?**

2. **What thoughts are you receiving back?**

The quality of the thoughts you transmit will determine the quality of the thoughts and experiences you get back through a process Napoleon Hill called 'Infinite Intelligence'. This is your own unconscious connecting with an invisible force that combines and communicates with the etheric intelligence of all the messages and information 'out there' in the universe. In other words, it's the theory that everything you need to know is available to you via something you can 'tune into'. This is commonly known as the 'sixth sense'.

Positive Versus Negative Thinking

Have you ever noticed how some people seem to attract bad luck? You can bet that almost *every* thought they have is negative in nature – blaming something or someone, or feeling sorry for themselves. They are stuck on the same frequency and the more negativity they put out the more of the same they get back. They often suffer physically too, as their bodies take on the negativity to generate illness or disease.

On the other hand, positive people are seen as having better luck: they attract good things and opportunities just seem to land in their laps. Born with the same potential as anyone else, a positive thinker can go from the humblest of beginnings (as in the case of Andrew Carnegie) and by a process of positive thought – combined with desire, persistence, planning and actions – achieve anything they want. Did Andrew Carnegie have any bad luck along the way? Of course he did! He made mistakes just like anyone else does, but he learnt from them and moved on – quickly. He looked for solutions, he learnt to think laterally, and most importantly, differently. Eventually, he found a process that created a lifelong philosophy for him and through Napoleon Hill, he shared it with anyone who cares to read it – and everyone should.

If you could meet someone who knew Carnegie or Hill, you would not hear them described as 'a moaner' or as a person who was 'always complaining'. That kind of SHIT thinking was not in their philosophy. Instead, they developed a strong communication with their unconscious minds through the power of autosuggestion and self-hypnotic language. These techniques enabled them to develop a clear and definite purpose for what they wanted to achieve, and then to devise a strategy to achieve it.

Say What You Want

Self-hypnotic language and autosuggestion are highly effective ways of communicating with yourself. Let me explain a little about how they work. We can think of our brainwaves as a little like tuning a radio or transmitter; depending on the frequency, we can send or receive different signals or information that can't be transmitted on any another frequency or level. For example, when you tune your TV into the History Channel, you can't expect to get MTV, and vice versa. By choosing to put ourselves on the right frequency, or in the 'right state', we can receive or transmit precisely what we choose.

We know that our brainwaves vary at different times in our growth and development, and in different physical states. This can be measured clearly on an EEG, which records the electrical activity of the brain. When we undergo hypnotherapy for example, the therapist aims to induce a 'trance state' by reducing our brainwaves to a lower vibration, or frequency, because this is where we are at our most suggestible and receptive. Our brains are operating almost constantly at this lower frequency from birth to the age of six, then less so to the age of 12 and even less often when we reach adulthood. This explains why children can pick up new skills so quickly while adults often find it more difficult to learn new things.

If you received *negative* messages from your parents or peers at this critical time in your life – i.e. when you were in your most receptive 'state' – you were more likely to accept them as valid and incorporate them into your thinking and belief system, where they dictated your future behaviours. Conversely, if you received *positive* messages, or constant praise and encouragement, during this formative time, it is likely that you developed a totally different, and more positive outlook, self-esteem and belief system. Your childhood environment, whatever it was like, had a profound effect on how you think and feel today.

When I think of this, I'm always reminded of Jodie Foster who, in an Oscar acceptance speech, thanked her parents for all the encouragement they'd given her as a child. She said they had made her feel as if 'every painting I ever did was a Picasso'. How different might her career have been if they'd told her to 'stop showing off', or said that she wasn't very good at anything? The comments and encouragement Foster received as a child had a positive impact in her formative years and have stayed with her for life; luckily for her they were positive messages. Not all of us have had that experience, but as adults we can access a trance-like state and use autosuggestion and self-hypnosis to delete negativity and give ourselves the positive, affirming and inspiring messages we really want to hear.

Even if you had negative messages in your childhood, remember this: It is never too late to reject a negative suggestion. The moment you begin to think and believe it is not true, is the moment you negate its effects completely. If you no longer validate it, then it's no longer true. This is very important, so I'm going to repeat it again and after reading it, I invite you to close your eyes for a moment and take this learning deep into your heart and soul with as much emotion as you can generate.

It is never too late to reject a negative suggestion. The moment you begin to think and believe it is not true, is the moment you negate its effects completely. If you no longer validate it, then it's no longer true.

What Are Your Thoughts Tuned Into?

Any thought accepted with emotion while you are in a trance-like state (whatever your age) will create associations that literally hardwire you to behave or respond to stimuli in a certain way *every time* you are in that situation. Have you ever responded angrily to someone and then said, 'He/she really knows how to push my buttons'? Have you ever looked at a cake, a piece of chocolate, a lump of cheese or any food and generated a 'need' and a strong desire for it, even though you're not hungry? That's another button you created by combining a thought with an emotion – you created a synaptic pathway in your brain to repeat that message or thought every time you are exposed to the same stimulus. But it only takes an opposing thought, combined with a powerful emotion, to delete that connection and wire a new one.

A nerve is an excellent conductor of electrical current and so is the brain. When the brain's cells send messages to each other, they produce tiny electrical signals in the same way that a radio wave is a disturbance within a quiet or still space. If a thought is a disturbance in the electrical current, then we have a scientific explanation for the power of thought that can be measured (as in an EEG). However, it is the actions or behaviours that result from specific thoughts that give them their real power.

The Incredible Power Of Thought

There is a perfect example of the immeasurable and unseen power of thought. In a trial, patients are given a drug that is in fact an inert substance, yet they get better as soon as they start taking it. This is called the 'placebo effect' and its success is entirely down to the fact that people *think* they are going to get better. In his book *The Biology of Belief*, Bruce Lipton talks about the power of the placebo and gives the example of a study in which patients needing minor knee surgery were taken into hospital.

All the patients were put under anaesthetic, but the operation was only carried out on half of them; for the other half, the surgeons made a small incision where the needle would have gone, so it would look like they'd had surgery, but nothing further was done. None of the patients were aware of the study, but the results showed that there was no difference in the recovery rates between the two groups. In other words, those who had the 'fake' operation got better at exactly the same rate as those who had the procedure. The only explanation for this is that they thought they had been 'fixed', and that thought was powerful enough to generate within them a genuine physiological healing process. That thought literally changed the chemistry within their cells to allow them to repair and renew their knees.

In the many years that I've been helping people deal with how they think and feel about themselves, food, or a traumatic event, I've found that for this approach to be effective, you must attach *a definite and strong emotion to the thought* – one that is powerful enough to generate change, either emotionally or physically, at a cellular level. If the patients in the hospital study hadn't truly believed the knee surgery would be successful, it wouldn't have been. We really are wonderfully made, don't you think?

The placebo effect is very interesting and brings up another, much less talked about phenomenon – the nocebo effect. This is when people take on board a *negative* suggestion in such a powerful way that it actually creates illness and disease. If you consider that positive thinking can heal a knee as effectively as surgery, imagine the implications of being told you have something that cannot be cured. Perhaps being told that 'depression runs in the family', and that 'it can't be cured – you have to live with it'.

In *The Biology of Belief,* Bruce Lipton tells the story of a physician who gave his patient the diagnosis of a cancer that was 100 per cent fatal. It was no surprise to the physician when, a few weeks after diagnosis, the patient died, as predicted. However, a postmortem revealed a misdiagnosis – the patient's body showed very little evidence of cancer and certainly not enough to prove fatal. The belief that he had a terminal illness generated such powerful thoughts in the patient that he actually changed his physiology and killed his own body.

'The Miracle Man'

If you want to see an amazing example of the power of positive thought, then check out Morris Goodman, otherwise known as 'The Miracle Man'. Early in 2011, I was privileged to attend an event where he was a guest speaker. In 1981, Morris, then aged 35, was flying his plane when it crashed. He sustained terrible injuries, breaking two bones in his neck – C1 and C2. People rarely survive a breakage of *one* of these bones, let alone both. He survived the journey to hospital, where he and his family were given a bleak prognosis. Morris, however, had other ideas. Although he couldn't communicate at all, he could hear what was going on and he made the decision to recover. He also decided he would regain use of his body and be able to walk again.

Morris began a process of visualization and thinking that would eventually heal him. After some time, the hospital staff realized he was fully aware of everything that was being said and all that was going on, so they taught him to communicate using a system that utilizes blinking to represent the letters of the alphabet. The first thing he dictated was: 'I will walk out of here'. As the months passed, many doctors told Morris that his goal was impossible and that he shouldn't have these thoughts because he would only be disappointed. Morris rejected this negativity and chose to have different, positive thoughts.

One key milestone Morris wanted to meet was the ability to breathe without the aid of a respirator. He was told categorically that the nerves to the muscles that expand the ribs had been severed, and that for him, breathing unaided was a physiological impossibility. Morris rejected this thought, though, and although he didn't know how his body could breathe naturally again, he decided it would. Every night, when the nurses left him to sleep, he started to work with the respirator. Instead of being passive and letting it do all the work, he tried to assist it. At first, he managed for less than a second, but he continued, night after night, to put his mind to creating a way of breathing by using autosuggestion – i.e. by telling himself with absolute belief that he could achieve it. He spent hours in a trance-like state, repeating that suggestion over and over again. After many weeks, he believed he could take a breath unaided and asked the staff to let him try. They told him it was not possible, but he was insistent, and so in the end they agreed, just to pacify him.

Against All The Odds

When they removed the respirator, Morris breathed unaided for over a minute. Everyone except Morris was stunned. The doctors kept saying, 'But it's not possible!' and whisked him off to a laboratory to find out what was going on inside his body. Their investigations showed that he had trained his stomach muscles to do the work of his diaphragm. After more training through the process of thought and autosuggestion, the respirator was removed altogether. It was a similar story with Morris's ability to swallow. Having been tube-fed, he believed he could teach himself to swallow, and he went about it in the same way until, of course, he could eat unaided.

Morris worked his way through all his body systems and his limbs, until, incredibly, less than a year after the accident, he walked out of the hospital. When he came on stage in 2011, it was the first time he'd given a talk for two years because sadly his wife had died. I can't imagine that anyone at the time of the accident thought Morris would outlive his wife – the family were told he wouldn't even last the night. That's the incredible power of thought.

Morris is the most moving speaker I have ever had the pleasure to listen to, and being in the audience was a humbling experience. During his recollection of his own experiences, he also told us the following story:

A man was loading meat into the freezer compartment of a freight train. As he loaded the last cuts, the door slammed shut. It couldn't be opened from the inside. The man shouted and banged on the door to no avail – the train began to move, making its long journey through the night to its destination. The man realized that he would freeze to death. He had no way of contacting anyone from inside the compartment, which was effectively a walk-in freezer, so scratched messages to his family in the ice on the walls. He wrote how cold he was feeling, that he was turning numb; his last message just said 'Goodbye'. When the train arrived next morning, the freezer compartment was opened and the man's body was discovered, along with his messages. However, the compartment had not frozen and the meat that the man had loaded was still soft and relatively warm. They checked the motor and found it was broken – the temperature was nowhere near low enough for someone to freeze to death. The man died because of a powerful thought that set in place the ultimate placebo effect – he'd thought himself to death.

As Morris stood on the stage telling us this story, a living, breathing example of the power of positive thinking, it was a painful reminder that the opposite is also true. Please visit www.themiracleman.org and view clips of Morris speaking. Since his recovery, he has dedicated his life to sharing and teaching the power of positive thinking. Usually, I think 'positive thinking' is a much-overused phrase, and one that most people don't actually register the power of when they are saying it, but when you watch this man speak, you truly see its power. If you, or anyone else you know, has ever been given a bleak physical diagnosis, then this is a good place to visit to show the doctors what the power of thought can really do. Doctors are in the medical profession because they want to heal, so they will be delighted if you can prove them wrong.

Your Brain As A Wi-Fi System

So, you know now that your thoughts are incredibly powerful things. You have been walking around with this loaded gun full of negative rubber bullets – probably firing at yourself more than anyone else. If you thought you were firing blanks, now you know that's not the case: *every thought counts*.

Thoughts truly are 'things'. They go outward into the 'ether' as vibrational energy, and they go inward to dictate your physiology: your physical, mental, spiritual and emotional health and wellbeing. When you put a thought 'out there' into the ether, where does that information actually go though? Napoleon Hill describes this space as 'Infinite Intelligence'. It's not a religious term – it's simply an acceptance that the universe is in and of itself 'infinitely intelligent'. Whether you believe the universe was created by God, or a force or an energy of such immense intelligence that it can actually manifest anything, including the planet, or whether you believe the universe was created by the Big Bang, the fact remains that the space in which we live – of which we actually occupy very little – has its own intelligence. There's even space within every cell in your body, so this 'ether' is also within you. It's like having your very own internal Wi-Fi system!

Exercise

When you make a call on your mobile phone, do you hear the words of all the other calls that are happening simultaneously around you? Of course not. Our senses are incredibly limited – dogs can pick up a level of vibrational sound that is beyond us; birds can see minute objects from distances we cannot – but just because we can't hear or see something, it doesn't mean it's not happening. As humans, we are limited in what we can see and hear, and many of us are limited in *what and how we think*, too. It's time to realize that you are the creator of your own limitations. Whatever you truly believe that you *can* achieve (with passion and a strong desire), you can achieve. What exactly do you believe you can achieve in terms of changing your body from fat to healthy? Write it down now and look at it. Is it what you want to and believe you can achieve or have you imposed limitations on yourself?

I truly believe I can achieve _____

_____

So, here's what to do with what you have learnt already (and in chapter 5, we will look at how you can use your imagination to do this even better).

You can direct your thoughts in two ways:

1. **Put 'out there' what you want to achieve.**

2. **Develop within you a thought process** that will direct your unconscious mind to a set of behaviours that will give you whatever you want, whatever the obstacles you have met in the past or meet along the way.

Remember, *every thought* has the potential to change the direction of your life. Have you ever seen the movie *Sliding Doors*? In it, Gwyneth Paltrow runs two parallel lives, each totally different as a result of one moment in time when she had a different thought. In one life she catches the train, in the other she doesn't. If you have seen it you'll know exactly what I mean. Her character is on the staircase going down to the London Underground when she hears a train approach and decides to run for it instead of taking her time and waiting for the next one. In one life she makes it, and in the other scenario a young girl steps in front of her, and in that split second she misses the train. Either way, it was the initial thought – 'run for the train' – that ultimately made the difference. Had she walked for the train, the second option would have been the only one. There are *always* choices, and there are always *consequences* to those choices.

Mabel's Journal

I tried a pair of trousers on today for work that I haven't worn for ages, and I could do them up! (OK, so I had my Bridget Jones knickers on – but it's a start!) I have definitely noticed a difference in what I'm doing, and how I'm eating, and what's really surprising is that I haven't even started the diet bit yet!! (I know I'm not supposed to call it that!) And I'm really enjoying thinking about what I am thinking about!

I really 'get' the concept of 'what you put out there you get back'. I know so many 'unlucky' people who constantly moan about their bad luck, then some more happens and they say, 'I knew that would happen.' Instinctively, I can't be around them for too long, and I understand why now. I'm definitely going to get together with other like-minded people and share some positivity! Think I will start a Facebook group!

Scary, the power of the mind. I've heard of the placebo effect, but I've never thought of it working in the opposite way before. The whole self-fulfilling prophecy thing makes more and more sense – you get what you think! After reading this chapter, I Googled Morris Goodman. OMG!!! Totally blew me away: the man is a legend. I am going to remove the words 'I can't' from my vocabulary – and if someone else tells me I can't do something, I'm gonna tell them to mind their own business!

Feeling strangely different. Two people at work today asked me what I've been so happy about lately... I said

I didn't know I needed a reason! Something must be changing though, because I actually went for a walk at lunchtime. It was a bit cold and I had to wrap up, but I quite enjoyed it! This evening, I wrote in lipstick at the top of my bathroom mirror: 'Thoughts Are Things'. This is to remind me to think about what I want first thing in the morning and last thing at night. Am getting better at visualizing; the image of a slimmer me is definitely getting clearer.

Here's what I wrote for the exercise today: 'I believe I can achieve... the body I want!!!'

Chapter 4

EVERY LITTLE THOUGHT HELPS

A common mistake that people make when they want to achieve a particular goal is opting for the quickest way of getting there. Sometimes quick is good – if you're a sprinter for example, then the fastest possible time is important! But if you want to achieve something meaningful and lasting, quickest is rarely best. This lesson is captured in a classic children's tale that we're all familiar with: the Three Little Pigs.

Once upon a time, there were three little pigs. The time came for them to leave home and seek their fortunes. Before they left, their mother told them, 'Whatever you do, do it the best that you can because that's the way to get along in the world.'

The three little pigs listened to their mother's advice and off they went. The first little pig, keen to get settled straight away, decided to build his house out of straw. He built it quickly and was pleased with himself. But the big bad wolf came by and when the little pig wouldn't let him

*in, he huffed and he puffed and he blew the house down;
and then he ate up the little pig.*

*The second little pig built his house out of twigs, but the
big bad wolf came along, and when the little pig wouldn't
let him in, he huffed and he puffed and he blew the house
down. Then he ate the second little pig.*

*The third little pig built his house out of bricks; he took
his time and his house was strong. When the wolf came to
the house, he wouldn't let him in. The wolf huffed and he
puffed, and he huffed and he puffed again, but the house
would not blow down. The wolf thought himself clever so
he climbed onto the roof to get in via the chimney. But the
third little pig was smart – he built a fire in the grate and
placed a large pan of boiling water on it. The big bad wolf
fell into the boiling water and was no more. The third little
pig was safe.*

The moral of the story is, of course, that the quick-
fix option, although attractive, rarely yields long-term
results. Sure, the first two pigs had a house, but not
for very long. And in the end their efforts killed them.
Extreme dieting can do that too.

A Modern Fable

Perhaps a retelling of the Three Little Pigs could go
something like this.

*A mother told her three daughters that now they were
adults, they must take responsibility for their own bodies
but that her advice would always be: 'Eat well and be
active'. The three daughters left home; they all found
jobs and led very busy lives. After a year had passed, the*

mother invited her children to come home for a family reunion. The girls had not heeded their mother's advice – all three had been eating and drinking far too much, and each had gained several stones and become quite fat!

The reunion was for a month's time, and the girls realized their mother would be disappointed when she saw them, so they all resolved to do something about it. The first daughter immediately rushed to the chemist for some meal replacement drinks and vowed not to eat until the weight was off! Overnight, solid food went out the window and in came 'shakes' in place of food. This daughter felt very tired within a day; she became lethargic, suffered from headaches, and had no energy to exercise. For fear of her mother's wrath though, she persevered for the full four weeks! She was rewarded with a weight loss of a stone.

The second daughter also resolved to do something immediately. She Googled the latest celebrity diet (after all, if a celebrity does it, it must be good!) and began a strict regime of raw vegetables and salads – no meat, no tea or coffee – with jogging and stretching every evening for at least 20 minutes. She was rewarded with a weight loss of just under a stone.

The third daughter looked at herself in the mirror and didn't like what she knew her mother would see, and what she'd say. She spent some time that evening taking stock of her life. She took a piece of paper and put a line down the centre. On the left she listed all the things she had been doing that had caused her to gain weight. On the right, she wrote down all the things she could do to lose it! The list looked like this:

THINGS THAT MADE ME FAT	THINGS THAT WILL MAKE ME SLIM
Too many takeaways	Planning meals to have after work
Snacking from vending machines	Taking healthier snacks to work
Watching too much mindless TV	Going to the gym 2–3 times per week
Drinking too much alcohol	Limiting drinking to weekends, and moderating amount
Not stopping when I have had enough	Having smaller portion sizes

The third daughter decided to make the food changes straight away. She went to the supermarket and filled her trolley with vegetables, fruit, lean meat, spices for stir-fry meals, nuts and seeds for snacks and a sports bra! Over the next few days she began to make some changes to her activity levels. She joined a local gym and began with a gentle programme to ease herself into it. After just a few visits she started to feel the benefits! At the end of the month, she had lost around half a stone. She also felt much fitter and more energized.

The day of the reunion came, and the three daughters went to see their mother. The first two daughters made a big deal about the fact that they had lost the most weight and that the third daughter was even fatter than they were! After the visit, the three girls left and went back to their individual homes, each vowing to continue with her new regime. However, the first daughter had tasted real food for the first time in a month, and it had reminded her of how good it feels to actually eat a nice meal! She decided to relax her regime of shakes only, and as a 'treat' for doing so well, she rewarded herself with a nice cooked breakfast. The second daughter also rewarded herself, with a Chinese takeaway, as a treat for sticking to her regime for a full month! 'After all,' the first two daughters thought, 'One meal won't make any difference!'

The third daughter went for a longer workout than usual the next day, to clear her head. The endorphins made her feel better: more positive and more determined. She knew she hadn't made as many strict changes as her sisters had, but she also knew she had to change the way she thought and felt about looking after her body. She realized that a step-by-step approach that didn't drastically affect her lifestyle, make her over-hungry or feel deprived, was the only way to do it in the long term. She began to look at crisps in quite a different way. Before, she had seen them as a treat, now she viewed them as harming and hurtful; they looked a bit like the nasty scabs she had on the inside of her thighs when her legs were at their fattest and rubbed together. She wondered why she had ever associated them with pleasure, when what they really brought her was pain – physically and emotionally. That thought empowered her.

The weeks and months went by. The first two sisters quickly resumed their previous eating habits, and of course began to regain the weight they'd lost. They didn't really panic though, because they knew they could get it off again any time they wanted by going back on the same regimes they had used for the first month. The third daughter, however, was enjoying her new life, her new body and her new energy levels. She found she was more productive at work and started to earn more money as a result. She became more sociable, too, and met a very nice man who had taken her out a few times. Her confidence and self-belief were rising and the weight was steadily coming off.

The next 12 months flew by, and again, the mother arranged a reunion. The first two daughters panicked: this time there was only two weeks' notice, and they had not only gained the weight they'd lost, but had each gained almost another stone! What would their mother say!? The third daughter had stopped weighing herself, but she had lost a total of four dress sizes since that first invitation 13 months previously. Life was good, she was fit and healthy, and loving life. She alone looked forward to the visit!

So, the moral of this story is this: if you want meaningful results that will last for the long term, then you must *change the way you think today*, but not necessarily expect great physical results straight away. I will explain more about this in Chapter 9, where I will show you how your hormone levels directly affect how quickly or slowly you metabolize fat and lose weight.

It All Adds Up

Let's say you are out for lunch with a friend who is about the same shape and size as you. He or she chooses Tuna Niçoise and you choose a pizza. Does that make you fatter than your friend straight away? Of course it doesn't! You think it's just one little choice that won't make you fat, and of course that *one* choice doesn't. Over the next few months, you meet regularly with this and other friends, and having eaten a greasy pizza and not got fat, the message is, 'One more won't hurt', so you continue to choose creamy coffees, pizzas and high-fat desserts, because hey, *individually* none of these choices matter, right? Wrong! After a few months, an accumulation of bad thinking and split-second bad choices really *do* matter. It's like compound interest!

Question: How did you get fat?
Answer: One bite at a time!

In his great book *The Slightest Edge*, Jeff Olson illustrates beautifully how every tiny thought combines to make you who you are. I believe this is true physically, mentally, spiritually and emotionally. *Every* thought counts. I have adapted this story based on Olson's teachings:

A very wealthy man was coming to the end of his life. Pleased with all he had achieved and accepting that his time to depart this world was near, he called his two sons to him. He told them he wanted to give them the opportunity to experience the full, rich life that he had enjoyed, and that he wanted to impart to them these three gifts:

1. **The first is easy to give and never runs out.**

2. **The second is easy to give, but not always easy to have. For some, it never runs out, but for others it constantly**

runs out. I give you this gift but whether or not you keep it is up to you.

3. **The third is impossible to give, but it can be gained. I have been showing it to you your entire lives, but I know not if you have seen it. I now give you an opportunity to see it before I depart.**

The man asked his sons what they thought these gifts were. After some deliberation, they decided that the first gift was love, and that this had been given and returned in abundance. The second gift, they realized, was the gift of money, and they acknowledged that their father had been generous to them financially. The father smiled somewhat sadly at this point, because his sons had not worked out what the third gift was. He lifted two boxes from his bedside table and opened one of them. 'I offer you both a choice,' he said. 'One you can make today, or in 31 days' time. In this first box is one million pounds. You can choose this box and have the money now, or in 31 days' time.' He then opened the second box to reveal a solitary, shiny penny. 'Alternatively, you can choose this box,' he continued. 'This penny, if you leave it there, will double every day for 31 days. I will await your decision as to which box you would like.'

The boys went to bed. One boy made his mind up before his head hit the pillow. The second boy spent a restless night thinking things over. In the morning, the first boy rushed to his father and took the million pounds. Within a week, he had interviewed and employed a team of financial advisors to help him turn his windfall into an even bigger fortune. They rented an office and got to work planning strategies for investments. By the end of the second week, the strategy was set and put into action. The boy left his team to it, because he believed his input was not needed. He decided to visit his brother, whom he had not seen for two weeks because he had been so busy planning his future, to see what he had done with his million pounds.

When he got there, though, he was astonished to find that his brother had taken the penny! He felt sorry for him because by day two, he had just two pennies, by day three, four pennies, then eight, then 16 and then 32. At the end of the first week he had just 64 pennies. By the end of week two, almost halfway through the 31 days, he had accumulated £81.92. The first boy told his brother: 'You must go back to father and tell him you made the wrong decision. That's what he is trying to teach us – that we must never be afraid to acknowledge our mistakes! He wants us to work it out and we have!' But his brother refused to go back to his father, and the boy was saddened by his sibling's misplaced pride.

By the time the brothers met again, over halfway into the 31 days, the brother who had taken the penny had accumulated a grand total of £655.36. His brother was horrified and again pleaded with him to go back to their father and tell him he had made the wrong choice. 'He will think we have learnt nothing if you do not go back and admit your mistake!' he insisted. But the second brother still would not go. By the end of the fourth week, the first brother's team had experienced mixed results with their investments; some had gone up, but others had gone *down. Even so, he had accumulated a profit of £500,000, taking his total to £1.5 million. However, when he deducted his expenses – wages for his team, commissions, taxes and office costs – he was left with £980,000. A net loss of £20,000.*

On day 28, the first brother went again to visit his sibling and discovered to his shock and surprise that the compound interest of the initial investment of one penny – doubling every day over time – had earned him just over £1 million! On day 29 it was over £2.5 million; on day 30 it was £5 million; and on the last day, day 31, his initial penny had become £10 million. And along the way he had gained wisdom as well as immense financial wealth.

In his rush to achieve success and instant results, the first brother had not stopped to appreciate the value of compound interest. The brothers had the same goal of course, but the second son learnt not to expect too much too soon, and that in the long term he would more than achieve his goal.

It's the same with our thoughts, and in turn, our behaviours. *Every* thought matters. You didn't get fat eating one pizza, one chocolate bar, one ice-cream, or one extra slab of cheese. You didn't get fat not going to the gym for one day or not moving any more than you had to for 24 hours. Your fatness is the result of the compound effect of all your thoughts and behaviours.

Doing The 'Write' Thing

While I was running my health clubs, I completed a Master's degree in nutrition and exercise science because I was convinced the more I knew the more I could help people. For my dissertation I wanted to look at the effects of food recording – of having to write down what you ate – and if (and by how much) this affected food choices. On the basis that to eat it, you had to write it down, I was pretty sure I would find it *did* make a difference. As students we had to follow and experience several different types of diet and as part of that process, we also had to record everything we ate for a set period of time and analyze the results. I certainly changed what I ate, purely because I didn't want to admit to the lecturer marking my work that I had eaten certain 'unhealthy' things. How hypocritical would that make me, as a student of nutrition and sports science. I wanted to be seen as virtuous!

So, I designed my study to run over 10 weeks and got a group of willing volunteers from within the health clubs, all of whom wanted to lose weight. I told them I'd be analyzing their diets, but I couldn't manage to do them all at the same time, so I asked half the group to record what they ate for the first five weeks, and the other group for the second five weeks. The volunteers didn't know the reason for the study, or what I was looking to prove.

As it was for a clinical study, it was important to remove as many variables as possible, so I asked all my volunteers to attend a nutrition course for an hour a week for six weeks prior to the 10-week programme. I asked them *not* to change what they ate over this six weeks, but to simply use it as a learning experience for the programme.

At the end of the 10 weeks, I analyzed my data and found, as expected, that irrespective of whether they were in group one or group two, the period when they *recorded* what they ate was when they *lost* the most weight. This was all good! But, in addition to that, I was amazed to find that when I looked at the measurements I'd taken when the volunteers signed up – i.e. before the nutrition course – they'd lost more weight over this six-week period than the whole of the following 10 weeks, when they were supposed to be making a more concerted effort to change their diets!

This was in spite of the fact that I'd specifically asked them not to change what they ate during the nutrition course and they'd all agreed! When I talked to the volunteers after the study was completely finished and I had my results, they all said they didn't think they had made any significant changes to their diet over the six weeks. But it was clear to me that they had made small, possibly even unconscious changes here and there, based on what they were learning about food and how the body burns fat. These small, non-deliberate changes resulted in significant weight loss for almost all the volunteers. These changes were little things that were so easy to do that they did them every single day and didn't even notice they were doing them.

You have to make changes – if you do what you always did you will get what you always got. As Albert Einstein said, 'Insanity is doing the same thing over and over again and expecting different results.'

The good news is that although the changes can be small, when they are repeated often enough they become hugely significant. I will teach you everything I taught my volunteers and more later in the book, and you can be even more successful than they were.

Mabel's Journal

I laughed out loud when I read the story about the three daughters. OMG, those first two girls were just like me (or like I used to be??). I've been down that road so many times, but I definitely don't want to end up like a dead pig! It's definitely a brick house for me now – no more houses of twigs and straw. I looked at the list daughter number three made, and was really encouraged. I think I must be on the right track, because her list was almost identical to mine! I like the stories in this book – they make it really enjoyable to read, and not too technical – and I find myself reflecting more and more about my own story. I wish someone would give me a penny and offer to double it every day!

I've now lost a dress size, and I haven't even got to the 'diet' yet! I'm changing the way I think, without really thinking about it. Not sure if that makes sense!

I had just one piece of my brother's birthday cake today. Was really pleased, because normally I'd have had seconds or even thirds! Felt really in control. Every time I don't eat something full of fat or sugar or other rubbish, I get a really good sense of achievement. I just don't want the pain those foods cause me. Didn't even enjoy the bit of cake I did have that much!

Chapter 5

'BRAIN JUICE'

A negative thought works in a stealth-like way; it goes unnoticed because of its small size, but it quietly combines with other SHIT thoughts to bring about a bad situation, physically or emotionally, or both.

Let's go back to the inspirational Morris Goodman. Do you reckon he thought sometimes, 'I won't practice my breathing tonight – one night won't make a difference'? Absolutely not! That SHIT thought would not have been allowed entry into his mind. He thought about how to breathe unaided *every* night, until he *could* breathe unaided by a respirator. He had a clear and definite purpose and a plan to achieve it. He thought about how to swallow *every day* and visualized himself doing it until he *could* swallow. He thought and visualized his limbs into action *every day,* until he resumed full use of them. He achieved all of this despite his doctors telling him what he dreamt of was not physically possible.

Doing It For Good

Let me tell you this now: losing weight is not a part-time occupation. It's a *definite purpose* in that you choose to focus your thoughts and your energy on the things you need to do, or change, in order to achieve it. By which time (just like the pig who took his time to make his house of bricks) you will have built solid foundations that will last and last. You will never stop wanting to be healthy and not fat, and your thoughts will never let you get that way again. Ever.

Unsuccessful people think that small, individual decisions do not matter. Successful people (just like you are now) understand the compound effect of positive thinking. If you change all the little things you eat, or the minor bad choices you make that lead you to become fat, then you will be slim. It's not rocket science, is it!? But it *is* a process: you must focus on how much you are *changing your mind* before you focus on how much or how quickly your body is changing. I promise you with all my heart, when you replace the way you think about food and activity with a more positive collection of thoughts and actions, your body will soon begin to show you the compound effects of those changes (remember the penny that turned into £10 million!)

The changes are easy to make, because they are usually very small things. But the problem is – it's also easy, if not easier (because it's what you know), *not* to change. You have to choose – that's free will. Other than your genetic skeletal structure, *you* get to choose the size and shape of your body. So which shape do you choose:

fat – or slim and healthy? Think carefully because there are consequences to either option.

The Brain Juice Diet

Your brain uses different chemicals to generate different moods or feelings. Let's call this chemical cocktail 'brain juice'. By training your mind you can literally change your brain juice to change how you think and feel and, as a result, behave. To illustrate the point, let's look at how our brain juice affects hunger and what actually causes some people to compulsively overeat. Always keep in mind that hunger is a primitive survival instinct that makes us seek food. Remember also that we still have the same genetic make-up that we had when we were hunter-gatherers and had to forage for food. Our chemistry and physiology have not yet adapted to the fact there's a supermarket on almost every corner and food is available 24/7. The process of generating an action to seek food occurs within your brain's chemistry (or brain juice): it is altered in response to internal signals from your body, and from external stimuli in your environment.

Your hunter-gatherer ancestors didn't sit on a rock watching hefalumps go by and say, 'Ooh, I fancy one of those, with large fries!' They hunted what was available, *when* it was available. Overeating didn't exist. Theirs was a hugely physical lifestyle, so inactivity was not an option either. You won't find cave paintings depicting your fat ancestors: obesity didn't exist.

If you consciously restrict your food intake to the point of starvation, your survival instinct will eventually kick in and, just as you cannot ignore the need for sleep, eventually you *will* eat. This is what happens, to a lesser extent, when you follow a strict, low-calorie regime; it's like surviving on two–three hours of sleep instead of the required seven or eight – you can do it for a while, but there's a tipping point at which your body demands sleep. If you semi-starve yourself with strict calorie restrictions, then at some point your unconscious mind will take over and drive you to eat. This drive is so strong it often causes bingeing and the feeling of gratification is then so great that extreme pleasure is associated with bingeing.

You have already learnt, and will read again repeatedly, how important associations are when it comes to creating behaviours. Remember the illustration of the iceberg on p.26. Have a look at it again now, as it clearly shows how experiences, when combined with strong emotions = behaviours. One extremely emotional event can be all it takes to create an association powerful enough to generate a behaviour that can be triggered over and over again, any time you are in the same situation.

Many overeaters think about food almost all the time; they are constantly on full alert for supplies! This is an exaggerated survival response. It's a bit like a phobia, which is a normal, rational fear that has been amplified out of all logical proportions. Your conscious mind tells you *logically* that the spider/cat/dog won't hurt you, but in your imagination you create an alternative reality that triggers a specific physiological fight or flight response – a change in your brain juice. A compulsive eater has the same exaggerated process in response to the need for food. When people constantly or regularly overeat, they think about food and what they could/should/would like to eat, pretty much all the time – except when they are actually eating. Ironically, when actually eating, they often just shovel the food in, sometimes even deleting the tastes and textures in their rush to get the satisfaction of having eaten it, and that brings temporary relief. This is an important point so I'll say it again:

It's not a specific food you crave, it's the feeling that food gives you. You are craving a feeling – not a food.

This happens through a mixture of the basic primal need for food, and the internal associations and anchors you associate with the food.

The Brain Juice Cocktail

Of course, there are many chemicals that make up our brain juice, but this is not intended to be a biology book so I won't go into all of them! It's helpful, though, to look at the two most significant chemicals that are associated with cravings (whether it be for food, drugs or even gambling), because it will become clear to you why you have certain feelings and responses. These chemicals are dopamine and serotonin. We need both in different situations, and they work in opposition to each other, countering each other's actions to achieve balance.

1. **Dopamine** – This chemical is involved in numerous bodily functions, including balancing hormones, blood flow

and the intestinal process of digestion. It is a survival hormone that increases alertness, and our ability to focus and process information. In an emergency, it can even be converted into adrenaline.

2. **Serotonin** – This works in the opposite way: it decreases our alertness and aids relaxation. When serotonin levels fall too low we can become irritable and can easily be overwhelmed by every day stressors. High dopamine and low serotonin creates the perfect environment for cravings and other compulsive behaviours. A rapid intake of carbohydrates can temporarily raise serotonin levels, but in the long term, this actually inhibits regular serotonin production. So, despite the quick fix, carbohydrate binges have long-term negative consequences. Good-quality proteins contain tryptophan – a large amino acid that converts to serotonin in the brain, stimulating natural and balanced serotonin levels. A diet too high in protein, however, can inhibit serotonin production. It's all about balance. (More about how to achieve this later; I have done all the working out for you and put it into the colour code system you'll find in chapter 12.)

Why Do We Overeat?

Hunger and the drive to eat is a naturally occurring process. In fact, it's lifesaving. So why does eating, or more specifically overeating, become an issue with some people and not others? It's all down to brain juice and the process of learned associations. When a slim person looks at a fat person and watches them eat when they are not hungry, they can't understand it. They say things like, 'If she really wanted to be slim, she would just eat less.' But it's not quite as easy as that – not without some mind-aerobics and some good techniques.

Think of a newborn baby. Its brain receives an internal signal that food/energy levels are running out and need to be replenished. The baby gets a signal that it can't consciously process as words, but it gets a feeling that means, 'I want food'. This creates an unpleasant physical sensation, or pain, that causes the baby to cry. Mum hears this cry and her breasts, full of milk, swell in response to its cry. She feeds baby and both are satisfied and relieved of the pain – and at the same time, a strong emotional bond is formed. Food brings a relief from pain. That is one of the key drivers of all behaviour – the avoidance of pain. Baby learns that when it sees or smells Mum, food is at hand and it anchors that comforting sensation with food and its Mum. Even if you were bottle fed, the process is the same – apart from the breasts! You are in pain, you get a hunger signal, you eat – pain relieved, positive associations made. The cycle is complete until the next time fuel and energy levels are low – it's a continual process.

Under normal circumstances, this cycle works well. But if you are a compulsive eater, a mixture of bad brain juice and associating pleasure with unhealthy, fatty, high-calorie foods means that the drive to eat is activated even when you are not hungry. Pain (not just physical pain but emotional pain, too) can also be a motivator to eat: studies have shown that when rats have their tails pinched and experience pain, they continue to eat, even though they have been fully fed!

Eating when you're not truly hungry in response to other factors (emotional, environmental or physical) is like any other reward-driven, addictive behaviour. It is no different to the gambler or the drug addict getting his 'fix' from his chosen poison. It's learned behaviour, driven by brain juice. In a recent article, Dr Steven Novella (an academic clinical neurologist at Yale University School of Medicine in the USA) discussed the historical ineffectiveness of 'dieting', saying that 'Research conducted over the past decade has demonstrated that the sensory experience of palatable food can easily override homeostatic controls of energy balance, leading to overeating in the absence of true physiological hunger.' This is a very academic way of saying that our thoughts can override our natural hunger/satiety signals.

Do You Think Before You Eat, Or Eat Before You Think?

For the first time, we are beginning to see a clinical approach to the understanding of what drives behaviour, and that obesity is a symptom of irrational behaviour that can be chemically driven via 'brain juice', and not a cause in itself. I am hugely grateful for this kind of research. For years, I have been working with people to help them change how they think about what, when and how much they eat and I have always believed the solutions lie in the head and not in the mouth! I have had to deal with all the fads, gimmicks and promises made by so many diets – high this, low that, etc. But I now have the technical material to answer many previously unexplained questions about why people overeat, so I can give you a complete guide to changing how you *think* in order to change your body.

Thoughts change your chemistry – emotionally and physically. They can literally change the cell environment so that it heals and repairs – or so that it fails and dies. *You* get to choose – that's what *free will* is all about.

I don't like the word 'willpower'. People talk about it as if it's a 'thing'. You must have heard someone say something like, 'Over Christmas, I just lost my willpower and gained three kilos!' Well, I have news for you – *willpower is not a thing*. It's not like your car keys, which you put down somewhere and then can't remember where you put them. We have *free will*, which means we have the ability to choose our thoughts and behaviours. That is never, ever lost. I've heard many failed dieters blame their lack of success on their lack of willpower – as if it was nothing to do with them! That's a cop out based on denial and deletion of fact. Whether you succeed or not is entirely down to the choices *you* make – you can't blame anyone or anything else.

When you change your mental state you automatically change your physiological state. You produce different chemicals in the fluid in and around your brain. How about changing your thinking to lose weight?

Get Juicing

To generate new brain juice, you must generate new thoughts. You must become a thought chemist. Just like a chemist blends different substances together to create a beautiful new perfume, you must now begin to experiment with new thoughts – and blends of ideas and beliefs – that will give you *a definite sense of purpose,* and a genuine faith in the fact that you will achieve your physical goals. Not can – *will!*

Faith is an essential ingredient in the process of permanent change. I am not talking about a religious faith, I am talking about faith as being a level of knowing, much deeper than belief. Dictionary definitions of faith include: 'Confident belief in the truth, value, or trustworthiness of a person, idea, or thing' and 'Belief that does not rest on logical proof or material evidence.'

When I think of faith, I'm reminded of a scene in one of the *Indiana Jones* movies where Indiana Jones has to reach a cup containing the magic potion necessary to save his father. He can see it across a great divide between the rocks and he has a 'clue' that requires him to 'Step out in faith and the path will appear'. He takes this literally and, as he steps out in complete faith across the chasm, a bridge appears beneath his feet and takes him across the divide. This is the kind of faith *you* must develop in your own ability to achieve your goal. You must step out and allow the bridge to appear – you might be surprised by how brave you are!

To develop faith you must first create a clear and definite image of you having achieved your goal. You must manifest this image every day until you can see it clearly in your mind. Please don't tell me you can't do this! You might not be able to at the first attempt – Morris Goodman didn't take his first unaided breath at the first attempt either, but he kept going until he got what he wanted! Every time you find yourself saying, 'I can't', you need to tell yourself to 'Shut the hell up!' 'I can't' really is a pathetic phrase when you think about it: now you really know the power of thought, use what you have learnt to get what you want. After all, that's why you're reading this book, is it not?

Exercise

Create a strong image of yourself as slim and healthy, and as already having achieved your goal. Generate this image first thing in the morning, as soon as you wake up, and visualize it throughout the day. See a successful 'you' popping up here and there. Focus on this image last thing at night, before you go to sleep. *Do not underestimate* the power of this manifestation of your successful image – it's one of the most important steps in the process of change, if not *the* most important.

Visualization is crucial for the generation of faith in your ability to succeed. Up until now you may have had a level of belief that said you'll always be fat and you should accept it. This is likely to be in response to other people's SHIT thoughts, as well as your own. To change it you need a powerful system to overwrite it, and that comes from within you. Instead of SHIT thoughts, **OPT** instead for **O**verwhelmingly **P**ositive **T**houghts.

Please choose one of the following options: Tick the relevant box:

1. Keep generating the same Self-Harming Invasive Thoughts – **SHIT** thoughts

   Yes ☐ No ☐

2. **OPT** in to creating new Overwhelmingly Positive Thoughts

   Yes ☐ No ☐

If you ticked yes to option 1 – you are *not authorized* to read beyond this point. There is no point. If you ticked **OPT**ion 2, you can now begin to use the process of visualization to develop faith in your ability. Not just to lose weight, but to achieve anything you set your mind to.

The Magic Of Autosuggestion

When you truly convince your unconscious mind of your genuine and deep desire for a healthy, slimmer body, you create a strong *definiteness of purpose.* You have now begun the process of autosuggestion or self-hypnosis, which will change how you think and feel about food for good. Your unconscious will begin to drive your behaviours automatically toward that goal. However, it is important to keep in mind that you are always at the steering wheel! There is no such thing as autopilot when it comes to achieving a goal; you must actively participate in achieving it every day. When you do achieve it, then you can go on to autopilot to stay on track – as long as you install an early warning system!

People are sometimes uncomfortable with the word 'hypnosis'; even the term self-hypnosis can unsettle some people. This is entirely due to a misunderstanding of the concept of being in a suggestive state, or 'trance'. We have explored the fact that you have two minds – a conscious mind and an unconscious one – and that your unconscious contains all the 'data' from every experience you have ever had, which it orders and files to create your beliefs and values and, ultimately, to generate your habitual behaviours. Whether you like it or not, much of that information was gained when you were in a trance, or a hypnotic state.

Many people believe that hypnosis is a form of unconsciousness resembling sleep, but in fact hypnotic subjects are fully awake (even though they may have their eyes closed). They are focusing attention specifically on their internal thoughts around what they are seeing (in their imagination) or hearing (self-talk or another voice). This 'focused concentration' brings with it a corresponding decrease in peripheral awareness, sometimes to the extent that the individual relaxes deeply physically.

This can enhance the physicality of the experience, but is not essential for 'hypnosis' to take place. In this state of heightened awareness of internal thoughts, we are highly responsive to accepting suggestions. In fact, this happens to you every day in conversation with other people, and you probably aren't even aware of it. It's the basis for almost every marketing strategy ever devised!

Lost In A Trance

Let's look at the occasions in your everyday experience when you may have been in a 'wide awake' hypnotic state. Have you ever been to a live music concert where the whole audience was totally carried away and immersed in the music? One thing is common to all the really successful bands or performers, and that is the ability to 'trance out' thousands of people at once. A few years ago I went to see David Bowie. It was the best live performance I have ever seen, bar none. He literally had the crowd eating out of his hand – Wembley Stadium was packed to the rafters, and all eyes were focused on one person and what he was saying/singing. More recently I went to see Kylie Minogue, who, with a completely contrasting style, also had the crowd hanging on to her every word.

On both occasions, it was mass hypnosis on a grand scale, and the performers inducing the trance were also totally hypnotized – by their audience. If you've ever been so completely immersed in a book or a TV programme that you block out your surroundings, then you have experienced self-hypnosis, or trance. Have you ever driven somewhere and then wondered how you got there? That's another example of an everyday trance.

In the past, hypnosis has had a bad press. Some of the stage hypnotists who get people to imagine they are famous rock stars and then have them 'perform' to the crowd have been criticized for using the technique. But you must trust your unconscious in that it will *only* allow you to do things, or behave, in a way that is in line with your beliefs. The people who jump around the stage impersonating Tina Turner or Tom Jones are often really quiet types – the reality is that some part of their unconscious sees other more extrovert characters doing things they might like to try, if only they had the 'courage'. By volunteering for stage hypnosis they are giving themselves the chance to be free from their limitations for a few minutes, and to experience something new. That is a conscious choice; they will be fully aware at all times of what is going on, and unless their unconscious is totally in agreement, they will not go along with it.

If you have ever watched a stage hypnotist you will see that he or she gives suggestions to the whole audience and then asks for volunteers to come up on stage. They will only select the people they have seen be compliant with the suggestions given so far to come up, though, and once on stage, the group will be whittled down even further. Those not fully accepting of the process will be thanked and invited to return to their seats. Believe me when I say that no one left on that stage is there for any reason other than wanting to be free of their limitations, if only for a few minutes. After the event they will have full and total recall of exactly what happened and even how they felt about it – they will laugh at themselves as they say, 'It wasn't really me!' but of course, it was totally them!

Walking Through Walls

There is a wonderful book called *Hypnotizing Maria* by my very favourite author Richard Bach (author of *Jonathan Livingston Seagull*). It tells the story of a young man called Jamie who goes to a stage hypnotist's show. Jamie volunteers when asked because he thinks it might be fun, although he doubts he can be hypnotized and says as much in a whisper to the hypnotist as he walks on stage. After whittling the volunteers down to just Jamie, the hypnotist invites him to take a walk 'in his mind' down some steps to a beautiful place. Once there, he invites him to open a large wooden door and go through it.

When the door closes behind him, Jamie describes to the rest of the audience the room he is in, which is made of stone and has no doors, but plenty of light. But when he turns around he notices the door he just came through has disappeared and now looks like the rest of the stone. Jamie is not in a trance, but he doesn't want to spoil the show for the rest of the audience so he decides to play along. The hypnotist then asks him what the walls look like. Jamie knows that they can only be cloth, painted to look like stone, as they have come out of nowhere and are some kind of trick, but in the spirit of the show he says that 'The walls are stone.' The hypnotist asks him, 'Are you sure it's stone?' Jamie then feels uncomfortable – he doesn't want to lie to the audience so he says 'It looks like stone, but I'm not sure', thinking that would cover it.

The hypnotist then invites Jamie to push hard on the stone walls, and to notice how, the harder he pushes, the more solid they feel. Jamie is a little worried about pushing on a cloth and pretending it is stone, but as he touches the wall it really does feel like stone. This is one impressive trick, he thinks. How has the hypnotist built a stone room on the stage without anyone noticing? He presses and kicks the wall, and it really is stone. He is a little frightened, but the hypnotist tells him not to be concerned, that there is a way out, and asks him if he can find it. Jamie thinks maybe he can climb the walls, as he can see light at the top. So he tries, but he can't get a grip against the smooth stone. He scratches the floor to see if he can dig his way out, but he can't, nor can he find the door. He feels foolish to have been tricked by the hypnotist, but he goes along with it anyway. The hypnotist again tells him there is a way out but Jamie still can't find it.

Eventually, the hypnotist says, 'Do you give up?' and Jamie replies, 'Yes!' He expects the house lights to go up and the mysterious, imaginary room to disappear, but it doesn't. Instead, the hypnotist says, 'Jamie, you can walk through the wall.' Jamie is shocked. 'I can't!' he protests, 'I can't walk through walls!' But the hypnotist presses him. 'Jamie, I'm telling you the truth,' he says. 'You have created these walls only in your mind – they do not exist, so you can walk through the walls simply by believing that you can.' The stone wall still feels cold and thick to Jamie's touch, though, and he starts to get very flustered. The hypnotist reminds him he is at a hypnotic show, that everyone can see him (he knows that of course – he's been playing along to keep the audience happy!) and that everyone can see there are no walls. He reminds him he has volunteered for 'fun' and tells him he will never, ever forget what he has learnt today.

'Help me,' says Jamie. The hypnotist replies, 'I will only help you if you help yourself. You must never be a prisoner of your own limiting self-beliefs. I will count to three, and then I will walk in through the wall behind you, take your hand and we will walk through the wall in front of you together. One... two... three...' The hypnotist appears at Jamie's side, takes his hand and disappears immediately into the stone wall in front of them. Jamie can only see his own hand holding the remnants of the hypnotist's arm. With a huge concentration of effort, Jamie follows and walks through the stone wall and back onto the stage... to rapturous applause.

Jamie never forgets what he learnt that day, although at times he forgets to remember.

The process of visualization, combined with emotion and belief, will change the way you think and behave – it will literally overwrite any previous programmes and create an unshakable faith in you that you *will* succeed.

Remember that your unconscious is *always* listening: it's like an internal 'Big Brother' who watches everything you do. Your unconscious isn't open to logical thinking in the way that your conscious mind is – it just acts on whatever information it receives – and it doesn't make the same kind of emotional decisions. It has a few golden rules however, and number one is to protect you! That means if you keep telling yourself dieting and exercising are going to be painful, and that you hate them, your unconscious will sabotage your efforts in order to protect you from the unpleasant experience.

Let me repeat that again more simply:

Be careful what you say – you are listening!

The flip side to this is that when you begin to hear yourself regularly saying (or thinking) that you are taking more care of your body, that you want to be slimmer because it means being healthier, that you enjoy eating new and different foods, that you enjoy moving your body more, then your unconscious will start to generate behaviours to support these statements.

Combining strong regular visualizations with on-going positive statements will definitely bring you the results you want. A key factor when it comes to visualization is this:

Your unconscious mind cannot tell the difference between reality and imagination mixed with emotion.

This means that if you genuinely experience some-thing, or if you imagine you experience something with enough feeling, both go down as genuine experiences and the information from them is stored in exactly the same way in your unconscious 'data files', which dictate your thoughts, beliefs and behaviours.

Imagination Is Reality

Have you ever seen a movie that was so scary that you couldn't get it out of your mind, or a book that contained descriptions or images that actually caused your heart to race? Perhaps you started to sweat or to breathe more heavily? How does this happen? You know consciously it's all make-believe, that none of it is real, don't you? The answer is that you imagine yourself being in that situation and how you would feel, and at that moment it becomes a 'real' experience.

In 1975, a movie came out about a shark that was killing people who were swimming just off the beach. The shark used for filming was made of plastic and rubber – in fact, for most of the shots they didn't even use a full shark model, just the front half because that was all that was in view – and the blood was just sticky, coloured liquid, and yet *Jaws* instilled so much fear in viewers that some left the cinema shaking and could never go in the sea again. In their imaginations, it was *them* in the sea, with a real shark, and it terrified them. Even a snippet of the famous soundtrack is still enough to make some people shudder with genuine fear. Such is the power of the imagination – it changes our brain juice.

This is *good news,* though, because it shows us that we can use our imaginations to create an alternative reality, and when we convince our unconscious of this new reality, it *literally* changes our behaviours to match it. I'm sure you have heard the term 'self-fulfilling prophecy'. This is when people talk about something so much that it actually happens. Usually this refers to a negative state, when people keep talking about and visualizing how they are not going to pass that driving test, not going to do well at that job interview or how their relationship will end… and then when these things happen, they act surprised, but still manage to say, 'I knew that would happen' or 'I saw that one coming!' For many of these people, the *only* reason these things happened was because they were directing their unconscious to *make* it happen.

So, now you have a choice. If every thought you have and everything you say about yourself and your ability dictates what will *actually happen to you*, is it worth a little effort to make sure you imagine and talk about what you *want* to happen? Or do you want SHIT things to happen?

Here's a challenge for you. For 48 hours you are only allowed to talk about the *positive things* that will happen in your future. If you think or hear any negative past memories, you are to reframe them immediately as a learning experience. Keep a record in your journal of your experience, either at intervals throughout the day, or at the end of each day.

Mabel's Journal

I always intended to try a 'juice' diet – let's hope this is more fun than raw cabbage and carrots! Janet keeps referring to Morris Goodman as an example of the power of thought and how it can change you inside, and I can see why. I wish more people knew about him – it would broaden a lot of minds, I think!

I laughed at the thought of our ancestors sitting on a rock by a cave choosing dinner from passing herds! It's hardly surprising that they didn't get fat when they had to chase their dinner; I get in the car to buy my meat. I don't even have to cut it up, let alone catch it. It's a bit of a no-brainer really. I'm beginning to realize how much of a carb-craver I was – I really did get the highs that come from what I now know is a serotonin rush, but definitely the lows afterwards, too. Good to know there's a chemical reason why I felt like crap after a pig out! (Apart from the guilt.) Not going to do that anymore.

I wrote 'I am worth it' on my mirror today. Then I put a bottle of L'Oréal shampoo beside it – just to remind me of what to think every morning and night!! Made me smile, anyway!

I _can_ do this!

The visualization is becoming easier. Have been visualizing during the day as well – kind of daydreaming but controlling what I daydream about.

Had a déjà vu moment when I read the Hypnotizing Maria story! I actually volunteered for a stage hypnotist a couple of years ago: I thought it would be fun! He had me miming and dancing to Madonna's 'Like a Virgin' as if I was her! I knew I wasn't, but at the same time I felt like I was! Weird. It was like it was me... but it wasn't me! I knew I was in control, and afterwards I felt really liberated. I wouldn't dance on stage as 'myself' but being Madonna really was fun. Could totally relate to Jamie's experience. I wouldn't mind being able to walk through a stone wall or two myself.

~~~~~~~~~~~~~~~~~~~~~~~

Tried something a bit different last night with my visualizations: I closed my eyes, counted back from 10 to one and imagined I was hypnotized into believing I could really achieve a slim body. Then as I was doing this, a slim me came into view, and I could really see her face and everything! I wanted to take a photo of her to keep with me, but I've been able to re-create the image, so I already have a photo in my head I can look at whenever I want. I then turned it into a movie instead of a picture, and watched her doing all the things that made her slim. Then I realized that I'm already doing a lot of them! Cool :o)

Chapter 6

MIND YOUR OWN BUSINESS

Here's a thought for you: start minding your own business. That means taking control of your mind to generate your own physical, emotional, mental and spiritual reality.

If you have a garden, or have ever been to a stately home with a beautiful garden, you will know that to keep it looking good takes effort. You can't just plant seeds and expect them to grow into perfect flowers – you must nurture them, clear the weeds from around them, water them and tend them regularly. If you do this you are rewarded with a prize of great beauty, a piece of creation that can be appreciated by all who come into contact with it. On the other hand, have you ever wondered why it is that weeds can grow extremely well with no nurturing or attention whatsoever? What's more, they suck all the nutrients out of the soil so the beautiful plants can't grow there; when beautiful plants do try to poke their lovely heads through the soil, they are quickly strangled and destroyed by the weeds.

Negative thoughts are just like weeds. If left alone, they will multiply and suffocate anything really worth growing. However, when they are pulled out, and more positive thoughts are nurtured, the rewards are immense. If we need water and specialized plant food to help plants grow, then we must need something to help positive thoughts grow.

Many self-help books advocate making statements and reading them out loud, but as you have learnt, words alone, expressed without emotion, are completely worthless. Writing a positive statement, specific to what you want to achieve, *is* a good thing, but you *must combine it with emotion* if you are to activate it. If you want words and statements to become part of your unconscious then you have to emotionalize them, otherwise they are just words.

This exercise takes practice – it needs constant repetition to develop the skill. Remember that Morris Goodman struggled to take his first breath with the respirator, yet within just a few weeks he was breathing completely unaided. You must be persistent, focus deliberately on what you want, and see yourself as having already achieved it. Make sure you do this every day. If Morris can teach himself to breathe, you can surely teach yourself not to eat rubbish foods and not to overeat – can you not?

Using Your Imagination

In the previous chapter you created a visual image of you having achieved your goal. Now we are going to add the words to that image that will create the reality.

If you want to do or achieve something, then it stands to reason that you should identify exactly what you must do in exchange. This is a level of understanding accepted by your conscious and your unconscious minds – it's the process of consequence. If you eat too much, the consequence is that you get fat and unhealthy; if you eat less and move more, the consequence is that you get slimmer and healthier.

Your imagination functions on two levels:

1. **Synthetic Imagination** – This organizes or re-organizes already produced old or existing data.

2. **Creative Imagination** – This creates new ideas and receives inspiration from sources other than known data. Connects with the sixth sense, both internally and externally, as 'Infinite Intelligence'.

Most, if not almost all of the time, people function using their Synthetic Imagination. Great achievers, however, function using their Creative Imagination. Alexander Graham Bell and Thomas Edison both used their Creative Imagination to solve many scientific conundrums and bring us things that we take for granted today: the telephone, moving pictures and light bulbs, to name just a few. Most successful entrepreneurs use their sixth sense, or gut instinct, to make decisions.

In the UK, there's a TV programme called *Dragons' Den* in which people who have a business idea present their concept or invention to the hugely successful self-made entrepreneurs, or Dragons, and ask for investment.

When you watch it you can see the Dragons elicit all the practical information they need and then combine this with their natural instincts before making a decision about whether to invest or not. You often hear them say, 'Something doesn't feel right about this deal – I am out.' They have learnt to trust their instincts.

Learning to tap into your Creative Imagination through the process of visualization, and attaching intense emotion and desire to your thoughts, is a fundamental skill in achieving something new.

Exercise
. . . .

Make a written statement outlining specifically what you want to achieve and by when, and include what you are prepared to do in exchange. It might look something like this:

'By 1 January next year, I, Janet Thomson, will have achieved a dress size 12. I will be healthier and I will be able to power walk for 4 miles easily without experiencing exhaustion. I will be energized and fit. In exchange, I will eat less, both in portion sizes and in the mindless eating of snacks. I will enjoy moving my body more through regular fast walks and trips to the gym. It's a done deal.'

It's important to include your name: remember *you* are going to be hearing this! Also, note the phrase, '*I will have* achieved' – this is more powerful than '*I will have* lost *x number of dress sizes*.' You have more positive associations with the word 'achieved' than with 'lost'.

Now it's your turn: _____

_____

_____

_____

When you are happy with what you have written, read it out loud. You must do this at least twice a day: first thing in the morning (learn it by heart so you can do it in the shower!) and last thing at night. If you do not do this one small thing, then you do not have the desire to change your mind and lose the weight! You are going to have to stay feeling like SHIT until you OPT for something better.

Do this exercise regularly, and your faith in your ability will grow and grow and the kinds of decisions and choices you make around food and activity will change automatically. As you learn more and more about how your body works and handles different foods by reading this book, you will already be deciding what changes you can make to your lifestyle before I even give you the specific guidelines, because you will have a *definiteness of purpose*. You must create a desire for a healthy body that is so strong that not achieving it is not an option. I bet even now, before you have got to the 'food bit', that you can already think of things and ways to change your behaviours so you lose weight?

Anchoring: Take Control Of What Triggers Your Behaviours

An anchor is simply something that triggers a specific thought – the exact *same* thought each time the trigger is pulled. It can be an image, a sound, a piece of music or a food. You are being 'anchored' all the time in your daily life. For example, most advertisements try to find something appealing and then anchor it to a specific product. Why do you think so many motorbike adverts show a scantily clad girl writhing all over the bike? It's to anchor sex appeal to the bike. If they showed some ugly bloke riding the bike, it would soon lose its appeal!

Anchoring is simply a strong form of association between a 'thing' and a feeling. In chapter 2 you learnt how thoughts become 'things'. And in the iceberg illustration on p.26 you can see that it's a combination of thought and emotion that creates a powerful association, and that becomes a behaviour.

Anchors can be positive or negative. If you've ever eaten a food that made you sick, then you probably don't ever want to eat it again – that's a negative anchor. Or perhaps a piece of music or a place brings back a sad memory.

Negative anchors can be used in a positive way, though, i.e. when you negatively anchor the foods you used to crave, perhaps chocolate or cheese, to the painful feelings you get from being fat that you wrote down in the exercise in chapter 1. If you strongly visualize and taste those foods while creating the feeling of shame/pain, or whatever you wrote, then your unconscious mind makes that connection permanent. Try standing naked in front of a mirror holding a bar of chocolate and saying to yourself: 'Chocolate did this to me!' If you combine enough painful emotion with the image, and the chocolate, you will create an anchor that will stop you eating chocolate. In the exercise below I have given you a 'craving crusher' technique that works on the same principle.

Creating An Anchor

You need to be in a 'peak' state – a state of intense emotion – to create an anchor. When you are doing this intentionally, as in the following exercises, then you need to be able to intensify a thought or association vividly in your mind, be fully associated into it, and then create the anchor at the 'peak' of the experience.

It may take a few minutes of concentration to generate enough emotion to be able to 'set' the anchor. Start to get yourself into the desired state, and when you achieve the maximum level you can create your anchor, and then reduce the intensity.

Exercise

If you want to stop desiring chocolate (or any other sweet, fatty or unhealthy food that you crave) you can simply anchor the taste and texture of chocolate to something disgusting. Then, every time you see chocolate, you remember this disgusting taste and not only do you no longer crave it, but it actually repulses you so much that you just cannot eat it.

Try this simple technique (note that you will be using a mixture of your Synthetic Imagination and your Creative Imagination to use the anchoring technique to change the way you feel about a food):

1. **Think of a food you crave**, but want to stop wanting (e.g. chocolate).
2. **Think of the worst thing you have ever tasted** – this needs to be something so repulsive that it makes you retch to even think about it. Perhaps you once ate something that made you physically sick? Now add to that some body fat scraped off the floor of a sauna at the end of the day, mixed in with some pubic hair from a public shower. Mix all these 'flavours' together and imagine how they would taste if you have them

in your mouth now. Close your eyes and take a moment to *really* do this, and when the revulsion is at its peak, squeeze the thumb and the index finger of your left hand together as you focus on the taste and the slimy, revolting texture. Imagine what it looks and smells like too.

3. **Create a mind blank by focusing on something different**, like a blue elephant for example, then repeat step 2. Do this at least 6 times until as soon as you squeeze your left index finger and thumb, you automatically imagine the taste and the smell, and see in your mind's eye the revolting mess and want to retch. You have now created a powerful negative anchor.

4. **Now think about the food you want to stop craving** – get a sense of the taste, texture and smell, and mix those sensations together with the repulsive mixture, so you have, for example, a chocolaty blob of someone else's body fat and pubic hair mixed together; use your imagination to really blend and combine the two until they are totally linked. Squeeze your left index finger and thumb again once they are totally combined in your imagination, and when the thought is at its most intense, blank your mind and think about blue elephants. Repeat this at least 6 times.

5. **Now imagine the food you want to stop craving** (i.e. chocolate) and if possible, get some in front of you to look at. In your imagination, see the body fat and the pubic hair mixing together with the chocolate and oozing out of it. *Really* see it in your mind's eye; smell it, and know it *is* there – inextricably linked with every single bar of chocolate (or whatever the food is). Now imagine putting that in your mouth: taste the body fat (this has a slimy, sticky texture

that leaves a film of fat in your mouth – much like chocolate in fact!) and the pubic hair, along with the food you used to like; imagine that it makes you feel sick. Really sick to your stomach.

Feel the disgusting mixture in your throat and squeeze the same left index finger and thumb together as you imagine needing to retch, because it is so awful – but make yourself chew and then swallow it and then really imagine you do feel even sicker. Taste the vomit. As you do this, squeeze your left index finger and thumb together again and anchor this feeling to this food using this physical signal. The idea is to combine the food you used to like and want to give up with the foods or things that are revolting, so your unconscious mind links them together forever. Every time you think about the food you used to like, you automatically associate it with this horrible experience.

6. **Now stand up and imagine** that a giant version of this horrible concoction is right in front of you (perhaps it's a giant bar of chocolate filled with pubic hair!). In a moment you are going to imagine it flying toward you at speed, consuming you with its revoltingness. You will need to take a deep breath in – and step through it. It may feel sticky, or heavy and horrible; the pubic hair may feel prickly and it may smell awful. When you have moved through it, feel it and sense it is behind you. I am going to count to three and then it will fly toward you, so imagine you can see it and smell it now: 1… 2… 3… POW!

Every time you see the food you used to crave, squeeze your left index finger and thumb together and remember to remember how violently sick it makes you feel; remember this moment. Use the finger squeeze to re-create it any time that you need to.

If you would like me to personally guide you through a visualization where you associate pain with old behaviours that made you fat, and then replace them with more positive behaviours and anchor some good feelings, visit www.powertochange.me.uk, click on the free *Think More, Eat Less* link and use the password 'Positive Attitude' to download 'Making Changes'.

Exercise

The exercise above is a good example of how to use a negative anchor to achieve something positive. You can also use a positive experience from a different situation to replicate a feeling of positivity. What feeling would you like to have that will help you to believe faithfully that you can change your mind and achieve whatever you want? Perhaps it's something from the list below, or perhaps it's something else:

- Confidence?
- Skill?
- Belief?
- Power?
- Control?
- A sense of achievement?

1. **Visualize how you would like to look and feel going about your daily routine *differently*** – eating differently and moving your body more. Notice how you feel. How strong, on a scale of 1–10, is your belief in your ability to make these changes? (1 is not at all and 10 is absolutely convinced).

2. **Now think of a time when you had this feeling in another situation or time in your life**. Perhaps you felt confident or had a sense of achievement when you passed your driving test, or had a successful interview? If you can't remember a time then *create one* in your imagination. Imagine that you totally and utterly nailed it – whatever it was. See yourself, in your mind's eye, looking and feeling indestructible having achieved something. Blend your reality with your Creative Imagination to create a vivid, strong image and feeling. When it really peaks, when you can genuinely manifest the feeling, squeeze the index finger and thumb on your *right* hand together. Or if you prefer, make a fist or some other gesture, to anchor that feeling.

3. **Blank your mind** – think of purple giraffes and then repeat step 3 at least 6 times.

4. **Now think about all the things you need to do to change the way you think about food and activity**. See yourself achieving your goals and all that you desire, and then fire your positive anchor. Blank your mind, think about purple giraffes and do this at least 6 times.

The more you use, or 'stack', an anchor the stronger it gets. Every time you successfully stop eating before you are over-full – i.e. you stop eating when you've had enough – fire that positive anchor off to strengthen it; to acknowledge feeling good about your progress. Every time you do some exercise or activity, fire it off again. You should be firing it off numerous times every day and at the same time seeing yourself *absolutely* achieving your goal. Staying fat is no longer an option – you have absolute *faith* in your ability and it is a *certainty*.

Your imagination is the control centre for how you change your thoughts and beliefs, and ultimately your behaviour.

Mabel's Journal

Been weeding out the last of my SHIT thoughts over the last few days – feels good. I used the 'Making Changes' audio download from the website and although it wasn't at all what I was expecting, I think it really helped. I listened to it for three days running and although I can't quite remember everything it said, I did do the visualization (even the unpleasant bits) and I definitely felt a shift – especially now I've done it a few times. I'm facing up to the fact that I was making myself feel like shit.

I've noticed I'm generally a lot more positive. Not just about what I'm doing to my body, which is definitely shrinking (got into size 18s today, without my Bridget Jones knickers!!). I am instinctively being drawn toward doing things that will make me slim. Sometimes it's like I can almost watch myself doing it and smile with pride as if it's not me, but I know it is!!

Thinking of crisps as being like scabs has really helped, because they actually do look like scabs!! Who would put salt and vinegar or cheese and onion on scabs and then bag them up to eat them!! Don't need willpower for that one – it's a complete no-brainer!

Here's my statement of intent:

'I, Mabel, will have achieved a dress size 12 by 25 December, and will attend the family's Christmas dinner in a sexy (not black!) size 12 dress. I will be able to power walk or jog for at least 30 minutes without stopping, at least three times per week.'

After I wrote that, I looked at it and thought if that's gonna happen, I'd better get my trainers out of the darkest depths of the cupboard. So I did, and then put on a fleece and dragged my arse out the door! So, I've just been for brisk walk around the block. Took 15 minutes and was puffed out, but I kept imagining I was walking behind a size 12 version of me – I could see it was me from the back. She was quite a way ahead of me and I imagined that I was catching her up. Really enjoying this imagination stuff!

~~~~~~~~~~~~~~

Following my walk last night I was fully inspired and buzzing at work today :o) Tonight I'm going to do the craving-crushing technique for chocolate!!

OK, that was a bit weird. I didn't think it would work, but I REALLY did imagine I was tasting chocolate mixed with slimy fish eyes (I tried them once in a Japanese restaurant and nearly puked!!), pubic hair and warm vomit. OMG! I cannot face chocolate now – I can see it looks the same, but in my head I know it is made of fish eyes and sick. Bloody disgusting! I can't believe I was putting that, and scabs, into my body almost every day! (OK, every day x 3!)

Chapter 7

ATTITUDE

I said earlier in the book that I don't know how long you've been fat, other than it's been too long, otherwise you wouldn't be reading this book. The reason for your fatness has been in your attitude – your attitude toward food, activity, and ultimately your body, and how you feel about yourself. How much you value yourself is vital in determining how much care you take of yourself. The L'Oréal adverts don't use the phrase 'Because you're worth it!' for nothing! It all comes down to your attitude.

Your attitude is ultimately the means by which you compile and then apply what you experience through a process of thinking. If each individual thought is a piece of your jigsaw puzzle, your attitude is the complete image it creates. It's what you see on a daily basis when you put it all together. Your thoughts create your image, and that's both a metaphor and a reality!!!

Napoleon Hill believed that it is your consistent, repetitive thoughts that form your attitude – they determine who you are and what you can achieve. He said: 'All thoughts which have been emotionalized and mixed with faith begin immediately to translate themselves into their physical equivalent.'

Hill demonstrated the power of positive thinking to create a positive mental attitude when a traumatic event happened in his own life. After Hill's wife gave birth to a son, the doctor came into the waiting room and asked Hill to prepare himself for a shock. He told him that his son had been born without ears and would never be able to hear – he would be a deaf-mute. Hill immediately told the doctor that he would find a way to enable his son to hear. For the next decade he devoted a huge amount of time to working with his son, trying to get him to respond to sound. He was successful and as a direct result of his unrelenting efforts, and his absolute faith in his ability to find a way, the child attained a level of functional hearing. He attended a regular school and was far from being a mute – his speech was normal.

When he was 25, Hill's son went to see a leading ear specialist in New York. After conducting a series of x-rays and examinations, the consultant stated that although he could see no evidence of any form of physical hearing equipment, the tests had confirmed that the young man had 65 per cent of the normal hearing ability. It was completely inexplicable and the doctor declared it a 'miracle'. The consultant also said he thought that, without a doubt, the psychological directives Hill had consistently given his son over the years had somehow activated a process through the boy's unconscious whereby he adapted and influenced nature to be able to improvise a reorganization of his nervous system. This subsequently connected his brain with the inner walls of the skull and enabled him to hear through a process that later became known as 'bone conduction'.

You Can Do The Impossible At Once – Miracles Take A Little Longer

The consistently positive attitude and self-belief demonstrated by Napoleon Hill and Morris Goodman achieved the impossible. Don't tell me you can't imagine yourself not eating chocolate, cakes, crisps, cheese, or whatever else you put in your mouth when you are not hungry because I don't buy it. Nor should you (the thought not the chocolate; come to think of it, don't buy the thought or the chocolate!).

If you were to interview 100 of the world's top achievers from a variety of backgrounds and disciplines – e.g. sportsmen, business people, teachers, authors, film producers, politicians – you would find a common denominator. And that common denominator is a positive attitude. On the other hand, if you were to interview 100 non-achievers from the same disciplines or backgrounds, you would also find a common denominator: negativity. The latter would probably be in the form of blaming others, or the circumstances, or just being unlucky, or in the wrong place at the wrong time, or missing the boat. The reality is that achievers experience bad luck and misfortune as often as anyone else, they just handle it differently. They chalk it up to experience and move on. If you have 'failed' on a previous 'diet' then stop blaming the diet and get over it. You learnt what doesn't work and that's a valuable lesson because you don't have to waste your time doing it anymore.

Over the years I have heard just about every excuse in the book for people's failure to lose weight. Here are just a few of the more common ones:

- I don't have time
- My husband/wife/partner won't eat healthy food
- It was Christmas/a birthday/a holiday that made me put on 7 lbs
- It's because of my job
- It runs in the family
- I don't like fruit and vegetables.

The list goes on and on. What would you add? Who or what do you blame for your fatness?

If you use this kind of language, then your attitude stinks! You are thinking like a fat person and you need to *stop* and start thinking like a slim person – that is a *happy* slim person. If you see slim people as sad and miserable because they can't stuff their faces, then that's a good thought to change right away! When you think about slim people, think about happy, healthy, slim people. After all, there are unhappy people of all shapes and sizes! Let's just focus on the positive ones.

When your attitude is negative, and you repeatedly make excuses for why you are fat, and why you can't get slim, you are justifying your behaviours and creating a powerful belief that will direct your unconscious toward maintaining that fatness. Everything you have learnt so far about your thoughts, and the effects of your thoughts, will have taught you that. You are already realizing that – am I right? So, now I am just repeating what you have already learnt. That's good. Good repetition is a very productive thing!

Exercise
. . . .

If you do want to be slim, you must genuinely and faithfully change your attitude toward your health and your body.

Write down the answers to these questions:

Where do you live _____

What does your home look like from the outside and on the inside _____

_____

If you have written about a *building*, something made from bricks and mortar, then stop and think again. You live within your own body!

Your Body Is Your Home

There is a very special and unique part of you, perhaps deep, deep within, that was created *before* you came into physical life – long before you took your first breath. Maybe you refer to this part of you as your 'soul', or your 'spirit'? Whichever phrase you use, this is your absolute essence, the source of who you truly are. I believe that not only did this part of you exist before you were born, but that it will continue after your physical body is done. But whatever *you* believe, know this for sure: there is a part of you that is not physical.

This special part of you – I will call it your spiritual essence – when connected to your physical body, gave you, and still gives you, life. What have you given it back? In return for these gifts, what do you give your spiritual essence? Unlike your physical body it doesn't live off food and water – it lives and grows, or shrivels and rots, based on the quality of your thoughts and your attitude toward the precious gift of life. How well do you look after the mystical and magical part of you?

There are many ways to look after it. The first and most important is to give it a nice, safe, clean place to live – that's your body. For the first few years of your life, this is the responsibility of your parents, but it has long since been your responsibility. You must accept that responsibility with a sense of gratitude, sincere commitment and responsibility. You can honour your spiritual essence by simply giving it a good home.

If you moved into a new house, of the bricks and mortar kind, and it was a mess – with broken windows, crumbling walls, and ceilings that looked like they were about to collapse – and all of this was visible from the *outside*, what would you do? If you would slob out and accept it and do nothing, then what are you doing reading this book? Most people who are reading this are much more proactive – they would not tolerate that kind of lifestyle. They genuinely want better things from life. They would refurbish and redecorate – or if that wasn't possible, they would move house. Am I right?

Magnetic Attraction

Your mental attitude not only affects your body, it affects every single aspect of your life, including who is in it. Positive people attract positive people; they can't and don't tolerate being around negative people. Take a look at who you spend the most time with. I once heard that you are likely to earn no more than the average income of your five closest friends. *Who* you spend your time with directly affects your attitude, because your unconscious mind is continually processing their shared experiences as well as your own. And because like attracts like (remember how your unconscious likes things that are the same), it's as easy to be drawn to people who have the same weaknesses as you as it is to those who have the same strengths.

I am not suggesting that you ditch any fat friends! But if you do have some then you must begin to protect yourself from their language and their behaviours. Create for yourself an invisible set of ear muffs that you can put on whenever they are moaning about this or that. Stop that information from getting through to your ears and create an invisible set of blinds for your eyes, so you can't visually process their continual 'fat habits'. Many children of parents who smoke start smoking themselves, even if they are told not to by their parents. Seeing is a powerful way of passive learning, which means you don't even realize you are doing it!

I strongly recommend getting together a group of friends or colleagues who have the same common goal of weight loss and health and working together to create a positive and strong group attitude. In this age of social networking this is so easy to do. Through Twitter, Facebook and other similar sites, it has never been easier to support each other in this way. You can also join the *Think More Eat Less* group on Facebook, where I will share my top tips and give you on-going support. You can also share your experiences with other like-minded people on the same journey!

Creating A Strong Mental Attitude

Your mental attitude is *completely* under your influence and control. You simply can't blame anyone else – whatever your situation. You only have to hear the story of Viktor Frankl to appreciate this. Frankl was a prominent and highly esteemed Austrian neurologist who, along with his wife and parents, was captured by the Nazis and deported to a concentration camp in 1942. He continued his work within the camps and prevented countless suicides. His wife was transferred to another camp, where she perished, as did both his parents, but still Frankl continued his work and became even more devoted to helping others. In 1945 the camp he was in was liberated by the Americans. As a result of his own hideous experiences and suffering in the camp

– and that of others – he discovered that even suffering has a meaning. He went on to write *Man's Search for Meaning,* which is an amazing and inspiring story of how a positive attitude can overcome literally anything or any situation.

A strong, positive mental attitude generates inspiration: it puts your sixth sense in touch with God, 'Infinite Intelligence', the 'ether', or the universe. Whatever your belief is, whichever word you use, it's the space that is within you and around you that carries within it and through itself information, and it is a source of power that you can access. You have your own internal receiver and transmitter, and your attitude is what tunes you in – or out – of the right frequency. When you are tuned in, and have a positive mental attitude, you can frame every experience as a potentially beneficial one, even if it doesn't seem like one at the time.

Recently, I was loading my car in preparation for a training seminar with a group of weight loss clients. It was pouring with rain. A guy who I had never met or seen before walked past me and had a right old moan about the weather, fully expecting me to join in with his negativity. He looked at me, waiting for a response, and I replied, 'Yes, but it's lovely for the ducks!' Completely baffled by my lack of negativity, the man stomped off. It was clear that he was used to being around people who feed his negativity in order to justify it.

Having a negative attitude is a bit like getting sunburnt on a cloudy day – you don't realize how harmful it is until it's too late. As Thomas Jefferson said: 'Nothing can stop the man with the right mental attitude from achieving his goal; nothing on Earth can help the man with the wrong mental attitude.' There's a great book by Will Holden called *The Guide*, which takes you through the process of changing to a more positive attitude in all areas of your life while telling a great story!

A positive mind keeps itself busy looking for the potential good in *every* situation. If you are going to a birthday party and see this as an excuse or a reason to 'go off the diet', view it instead as an opportunity to learn how to have a great time without getting fatter. Then view that as an opportunity to learn a skill that will no doubt come in very handy on countless occasions once you have mastered it!

Here are the steps to follow for creating a strong mental attitude:

1. **First, you must create a strong and intense desire for what you want to achieve.** This desire must become a passion, an absolute *must have*.

2. **Next, you must identify the thoughts and behaviours that have kept you from achieving this goal.** You need to know what you have to *stop* doing before you *start* doing something else, otherwise you are giving yourself mixed messages. If you are working on your computer and you want to delete a paragraph, you have to find the exact paragraph and highlight it before you can delete it. You need to acknowledge what you are deleting, and be prepared to let it go in exchange for having something much better.

3. **You must generate a clear, visible image or representation of you as already having achieved your goal**, and then generate powerful, positive emotions when you see it. This visualization must be repeated at least twice daily.

4. **You must add words or statements to that goal**, and you must repeat them out loud with passion and belief to generate absolute faith and to change your 'brain juice'. You must do this at least twice a day, with your visualizations.

5. **You must, through the process of positive self-talk, autosuggestion or self-hypnosis, constantly feed yourself positive statements** and directives to maintain healthy 'brain juice'.

6. **You must regularly associate with like-minded people who have already achieved, or are achieving, the same or similar goals.** The sense of belonging to a group is important because it creates a feeling of safety. This is a natural survival instinct based on hunter-gatherers being safer in groups. It can also positively affect brain juice. Make sure you have some positive and encouraging communication every day, whether in person or through social networks such as our *Think More Eat Less* Facebook page.

7. **You must continue to read and/or listen to audio recordings that will feed your mind with positive thoughts and suggestions.** Aim to do this for at least 15 minutes a day. This is easy to do because most of us

have MP3 players on our phones, or CD players in the car. Put something positive on when you are getting dressed in the morning, instead of putting the TV on and watching depressing news. Start the day with a positive *mental* breakfast as well as a nutritious food one. You can access some free audio downloads to help you change your mind to a more positive state at www.powertochange.me.uk. Click on the *Think More, Eat Less* link on the home page, and enter the password 'Positive Attitude'.

8. **You must develop knowledge and skills that will make achieving your goals easier.** In this case, the nutrition and 'how your body works' sections of this book will do this, but read and re-read the entire book over and over. This book will be at its most powerful when you are reading it for the second or maybe the third time. When you find you are already thinking ahead to what's coming next, you've got it! Remember, this is *not* a novel – you must read it all the way through, slowly and thoughtfully, and then do it again. And maybe again! It's a resource, and along with the audio downloads from the website, it forms the basis of *all you need to change*.

Mabel's Journal

I haven't read any more of the book for a week or so, because I've been reflecting on everything I have changed so far. Janet says at the beginning that it's not a novel and to read it at your own pace, but I have realized there's a big difference between reading it and <u>doing</u> it, so I'm going to make a more concerted effort to <u>do</u> stuff. Wrote this on a piece of paper today: 'The Mind Is What the Brain Does' and stuck it on the fridge. My brain is 'doing' slim!!

It's funny that this chapter is about attitude – as I read it today, I realized how much my attitude has, and still is, changing – not just toward how I'm changing what I eat naturally (I still haven't got to the diet bit!). I'm definitely moving more (have been for three walks this week and am a few steps closer to the slim me who walks just ahead!).

When I look back at my life and all the people who told me I couldn't do this or I couldn't do that, it occurs to me... what if they were wrong??? Where would I be if I had believed from a young age that I could achieve whatever I wanted (like Jodie Foster)? Thank God it's not too late. Thought for the day: 'It's never too late to undo a negative suggestion – especially if it's someone else's SHIT!'

If a man can walk again after breaking his neck twice, and if a man can teach his son to hear when he has no functional ears or mechanism to hear, then I can CERTAINLY change how I think and behave – and be slim! I can also be more confident in myself and get a better job – I'm fed up with settling for less.

Did the positive anchor exercise today. Not sure how well it worked, or if it will last, so I need to try it out. But it did feel really good when I did it! Remembered the day I passed my driving test! That felt really good because it gave me complete freedom and independence. Perhaps being slim will do the same???

Chapter 8

TAP INTO YOUR POSITIVITY

So far, you have learnt how your brain works, and some powerful techniques to change how you think and feel. Now I am going to show you an exciting and very simple therapy that you can use to eliminate, or 'collapse', negative feelings, such as cravings or lack of motivation. It's called Thought Field Therapy (TFT). My last book, *Tapping For Life* (Hay House, 2009), explains more fully how this amazing technique works, and how it can be used specifically to collapse negative emotions, anxiety and past traumas, but this chapter offers a brief overview of the technique, specifically how to stay positive and eliminate cravings.

People often overeat because of sadness, or some upset in an aspect of their lives. Dealing with these issues, so they stop affecting them on a day-to-day basis, is invaluable – not just for weight loss, but in order to move on in a positive way. When people come to see me for help with weight loss, I often begin by removing negative emotions, anxiety, and even depression, and build self-esteem and self-worth before moving on to work on the issue of weight loss.

Earlier in the book we explored the fact that when people eat when they are not hungry, it's to get a *feeling*. Often, it's to get *any* feeling other than the one they are experiencing, and they seek solace in the sensation food gives them. They become *anchored* to feeling better when they eat. This is called 'comfort eating'. If you remove the causes of the negative feelings – whether it's a past trauma or anxiety, or a stress of some kind – the need to eat to get rid of that feeling by comfort eating disappears.

What then happens is that, as you start to feel better about yourself, you generally start to take more care of your body and you begin to lose weight without really trying. Changes that do need to be made become easier, because you know you really are worth the effort.

How TFT Works

TFT is essentially an energy therapy that works by using the meridians – the invisible energy pathways used for centuries in traditional Chinese medicine, particularly in acupuncture. The Chinese identified the meridians as pathways that work like a circuit, flowing and conducting energy throughout the body. They believe that we store an imprint of our emotions within these pathways and that they are the link between the emotional mind and the body. It might be helpful to think of the meridians as 'emotional highways' or roads. If there's a crash on a road, it creates a blockage and traffic cannot flow. In the same way, a trauma or anxiety can cause a blockage in your meridians that prevents energy from flowing, causing emotional or physical distress, or both.

The developer of the technique of TFT, American psychologist Dr Roger Callahan, discovered that these blockages can be cleared by tapping on very specific points. Whereas an acupuncturist would insert a needle, with TFT you simply 'tap' the same spot. You can do TFT on yourself – there are absolutely *no* harmful side effects and even if you do it wrong, it doesn't matter. It won't work, but you will do yourself absolutely no harm at all; it the safest of all therapies.

Your body has a polarity. This can be tested using a standard electrician's volt-meter, which can measure positivity and negativity. When you are 'positive', cells can function normally and the process of growth and repair can take place naturally. When the cells' polarity is negative, however, healing and regeneration cannot take place. Imagine the battery in your TV remote being put in upside-down – the remote just won't work until you change it around to get the positive connection. Your body is the same. What is important is that negativity as measured in terms of polarity also affects us emotionally. When you are in a negative state all negative emotions are amplified – fears, cravings, and all negative thoughts become more powerful and consuming.

In TFT this state is called 'Psychological Reversal', which is when your thoughts are the exact *opposite* of how you would like to feel – i.e. negative instead of positive. When you are 'reversed' you are prone to self-sabotage in your thoughts and your behaviours. You can correct this by changing your state and your physiology – in other words your 'brain juice'. Exercise, and the generation of endorphins, can correct the imbalance, but it's not always practical to put on some lively music and dance around laughing to generate an endorphin boost! Thankfully, TFT offers us a simpler way of restoring the correct balance – it's called the TFT Triangle. Through tapping on very specific meridian points that literally balance the body's energy, it can return us to 'positivity'.

The TFT Triangle

If you have a negative thought, simply hold that thought and, using two or three fingers of one hand, tap on the following points firmly but not too hard for about 10 seconds each.

1. **Side of hand (sh)**   2. **Index finger (if)**

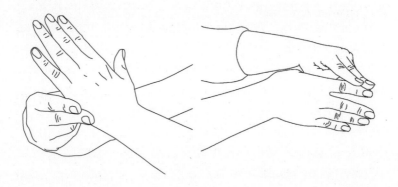

3. Under nose (un)

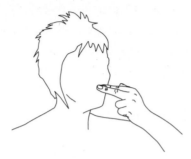

4. Under lip (ul)

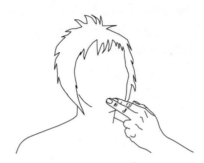

5. Repeat under nose (un)

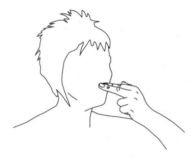

6. Index finger other hand (if)

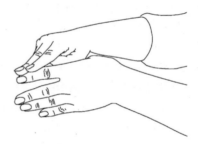

7. Side other hand (sh)

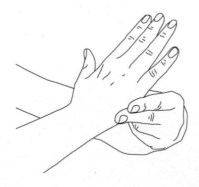

This sequence is called the 'triangle' because you start with one hand, work up to the face, then work down to the other hand, making a triangle shape. Tapping can be used to remove any negative thought or feeling. You can use the 'triangle'

to collapse negativity, but it is also important to prevent negativity *before* it occurs, too, so get into the habit of doing the sequence every morning as you are doing your visualizations, and every evening before you go to sleep as you are doing your visualizations. This will ensure that the images are positive. I do the triangle every morning in the shower and every evening after I've cleaned my teeth. I also do it any time I get a negative or irrational thought, or when I just feel I need an emotional re-boot.

There is another TFT technique that works especially well to collapse food cravings.

Tapping Cravings Away

Focus your mind on the food you crave – if possible, look at it and smell it so you are really 'in the thought'. Then rate the craving from 1–10, with 10 being a full-on craving and one being 'not bothered'.

Tap the following points for approximately 10 seconds each:

1. Side of hand (sh)   2. Under nose (un)

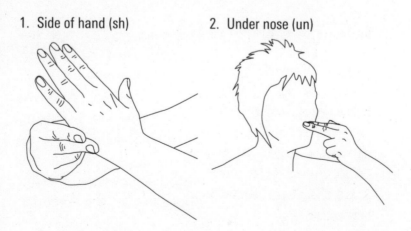

3. Collar bone (c)

4. Under eye (e)

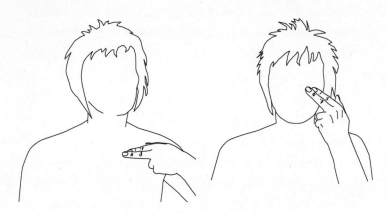

5. Collar bone (c)

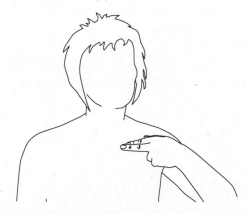

6. Then tap the gamut spot, on the back of your hand between the little finger and ring finger knuckles (see right) continually. As you do so, hum a few bars of a tune (e.g. 'Happy Birthday'), then count 1, 2, 3, 4, 5, out loud. Stop and then hum again.

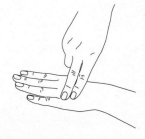

7. Still tapping, look down toward one shoulder, keeping your head still. Then look toward the other shoulder; then roll your eyes up and all the way round 360 degrees; then roll them around the other way.

8. Tap the first sequence again.

9. Now rate the craving on a scale of 1–10. It will probably have reduced. Repeat the entire process until the craving has gone. Then close your eyes and anchor the feeling of control you have established. Appreciate that you are not under the control of a craving, and that *you* get to choose what you put in, and as a result 'on', your body.

Combining TFT with the other techniques in the book, and of course the colour code nutrition system coming up, will give you all the tools you need to turn your life and your health around – for good.

Mabel's Journal

I've heard of tapping – a friend of mine had it when she became very anxious about driving after a car accident. Literally, after the first session she could drive again, so I already knew this stuff works. I'm going to teach her this 'triangle' because she has a few other anxieties that it might help with!

Got a really heavy weekend coming up – a family 'do'. I'm not looking forward to it at all and I have to make *a speech congratulating my auntie and uncle on their 25th wedding anniversary. I can't believe I got roped into that one! So I'm definitely going to try this technique out for that. Watch this space!*

~~~~~~~~~~~~~~~~~~~~~~

Well, the weekend couldn't have got off to a worse start! I forgot to do the triangle in the morning; my brother had overslept and wasn't ready when I picked him up, so we were late; he and my sister had a big bust up over the seating arrangements and it was pouring with rain all the way to the hotel. It took two hours to do a 45-minute drive so I arrived well fed up! Went into the loo at the hotel to repair the damage to my hair from running across the car park in torrential rain (I looked like a drowned rat!), and when I got my hairbrush out of my bag I saw the piece of paper with the triangle written on it!

Couldn't get any worse, I thought, so stood there tapping. It was weird – I literally felt the anger and frustration melt away. I did it three times, and found myself taking deeper breaths and just letting all the SHIT go! Did it again just before my speech and actually felt quite good! Wore an outfit I hadn't worn for ages, which is a size 18, and it was a little loose! Got lots of compliments and people kept saying how well I looked. If I had any doubts about the benefits of tapping I haven't now! It's four weeks since I started reading the book and 'doing' the stuff in it, and it is definitely changing something!!

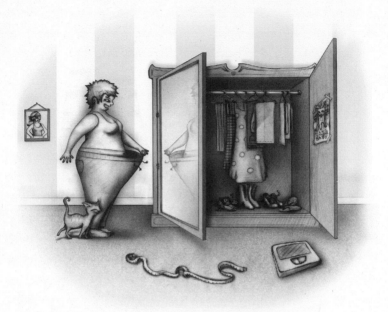

It's now Wednesday, and since the weekend I've been doing the triangle every morning, looking in the mirror, making my positive statements out loud and REALLY meaning them! Gives me a little boost every time and only takes a minute. Even did it before my walk yesterday and I'm sure I'm getting closer to the 'me' in front – I even jogged for a whole minute! Felt so good when I got back that I did my positive anchor again to reinforce it, and the sense of achievement was brilliant. In days gone by, I would have got back, told myself how knackered I was and how awful it was and wished I could have had some nice food as a reward! This time I got back, was automatically thinking about how much closer to a slimmer me I am, and had a good long soak in the bath. Feeling really pleased with myself!

Chapter 9

HORMONES R US

Here's the thing: you look at yourself in the mirror and think, 'I'm fat!' and decide that you really *do* want to correct this situation. In other words, to lose fat and be slim. The reality though is that the fat is just a symptom – it's your body showing you, and advertising to everyone else, that you've been treating it with disrespect and neglect. You've been eating more than you've been moving. The cause of this is a combination of your behaviours, and the physical and physiological effects they have on your body. You are 'wearing' those effects right now.

Step-by-Step Weight Loss

There are essentially two ways to lose weight, and to be successful now and forever you need to address both of them:

1. **Think More, Eat Less, Move More**

2. **Manage Your Hormones and Your Metabolism**

In this and the next chapter you are going to learn how your body can be turned from a highly efficient, fat-storing machine into a highly efficient fat-burning machine, simply by making some key changes to the balance of your diet (and without having to spend hours at the gym!). An unhealthy body is great at storing fat, but rubbish at burning it. A healthy body, on the other hand, is great at burning fat and rubbish at storing it. The good news is – you get to choose which way your body works.

The different systems in the body are interconnected and their combined effects give us optimum health. When it comes to weight loss, the most important systems, or factors, are those shown in the graphic below.

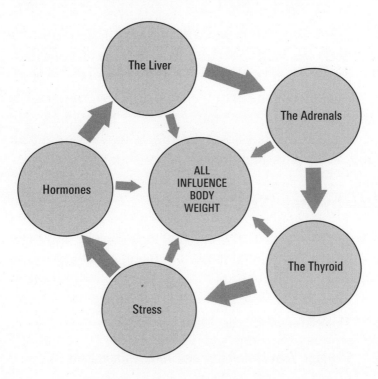

The Liver

Let's start with the liver, because it's arguably the most important organ when it comes to weight loss. When you think of your digestive system, you probably think of your stomach, your intestines and your bowels, but you probably don't think about your liver. Yet this key organ is not only responsible for filtering everything that goes through your body (just like an oil filter on a car), it also has a huge impact on how you metabolize and store food as energy – and how you make that energy available for use, as and when needed.

Although the liver is an organ, it is also considered a gland, because it produces bile. A poorly functioning liver can cause fluid to leak into the area just below the rib cage, giving a pot belly appearance. Unlike rolls of fat, this sac of fluid feels more solid and can actually be pushed from side to side. A dysfunctional liver is caused by a lack of nutrients and an imbalanced diet. Your liver will produce obvious physical symptoms if it is not looked after. As well as the pot belly, you may notice that your tongue looks white and furry and has a crease down the centre. You may have severe, on-going itching, pain in the right shoulder, liver spots, or a yellow colour to the skin or the whites of the eyes known as jaundice. People with a poorly functioning liver often suffer from bloating, especially after eating gluten, which is found in grains. The gluten in rice and corn is safe for celiac patients (who cannot tolerate even minute amounts of gluten), but the gluten in wheat, barley and rye is not.

More serious liver conditions include hepatitis – inflammation of the liver – and cirrhosis – a late stage of liver disease that causes a build-up of scar tissue. Although a dysfunctional liver can inhibit fat burning, and therefore weight loss, a severely dysfunctional and diseased liver usually results in drastic weight loss.

Despite all the symptoms of physical stress, an overworked liver retains an amazing capacity to perform its functions, which explains why so many people have advanced liver dysfunction before being diagnosed. If you think you may have the symptoms of a severely dysfunctional liver, go to www.britishlivertrust.org.uk for more information; if you are still concerned, consult your GP. If you think you may have some signs of a slightly dysfunctional liver, which may be contributing to your weight gain, then this chapter and the colour coded nutrition system in chapter 12 will show you how you can help correct it naturally.

What the Liver Does

The liver is situated on the right-hand side, at the bottom of the rib cage, and it is directly 'plumbed into' to the digestive system and the heart for circulation. It has many functions, including the following:

- Production of bile – required for the digestion of fats
- Filtering of hormones
- Converting the extra glucose in the body into stored glycogen in liver cells; and then converting it back into glucose for energy when needed

- Production of blood-clotting factors
- Production of amino acids (the building blocks for making proteins), including those used to help fight infection
- Processing and storage of iron – essential for red blood cell production
- Manufacture of cholesterol for growth and repair, and other chemicals required for fat transport
- Conversion of waste products of body metabolism into urea, which is then excreted in the urine
- Metabolization of medications into their active ingredients in the body.

A healthy liver is essential for effective, long-term weight loss but it can be stressed or damaged by several factors. Here are some of the key ones:

- Alcohol
- A high intake of sugar
- A diet low in nutrients
- A diet high in caffeine
- Long-term use of certain medications
- Smoking.

If you are serious about wanting to lose weight, for the next few weeks spend some time looking after your liver and the whole process of burning fat will become much easier. I will tell you specifically how to do this of course! And not only in this chapter – the colour code system in chapter 12 has been designed to promote healthy liver function.

Here are some foods that promote a healthy liver:

- **Cruciferous Vegetables**, for example, broccoli, cauliflower, Brussels sprouts, kale, cabbage, pak choi. These all contain vitamins, minerals and fibre. As well as aiding digestion and fat burning, they contain phytochemicals that can stimulate enzymes in the body that detoxify carcinogens before they damage cells, helping prevent cancer.
- **Foods containing sulphur**, such as garlic, legumes, onions and eggs.
- **Good sources of water-soluble fibre**, including pears, oat bran, apples, and legumes.
- **Artichokes, beets, carrots, dandelion, cranberries (and most other berries), turmeric and cinnamon.**
- **Good-quality protein foods**, such as fish, tofu or organic chicken.

As the liver is a detoxifying organ, it's important to maintain good levels of hydration to flush toxins out once the liver has processed them.

Constipation can cause liver problems because the bowel isn't able to excrete the toxins through the faeces, so they stay in the body and have to be cleared by the liver. Therefore a diet high in fibre is indirectly linked to the health of the liver.

It can take years of abuse to severely impair liver function, but once the damage is done, a good, detoxifying diet and a reduction in stress can rejuvenate this organ, often in just a few months. You are likely to notice a difference in energy levels and improved digestion after just two weeks of eating a vegetable-rich diet that also contains high-quality proteins such as fish and organic chicken. The colour code system in chapter 12 makes this really easy to achieve.

Exercise
. . . .

Think of three things that you can start doing *now* that will boost your liver function, and therefore your ability to burn fat. Now write them down – this is important, because it makes you focus, and it uses a different part of your brain than just thinking it. So just do it! When you have written the three things down, say them out loud to make a statement (you know from earlier chapters how powerful this is). As you do this, visualize these changes *actually happening* inside your body. Let's say for example that you write for the first one:

1. **I will make a cranberry and mixed-berry fruit smoothie every day.** You then say exactly that out loud and add at the end, 'And it will help my body to become healthy and lose weight'. You have to mean this as you say it, and of course, you know you must attach emotion to it. Each morning, as you drink your smoothie, say the words and then visualize how healthy the smoothie is making you as you drink it. In this way you create positive anchors to it, and you change your mental and your physical physiology at the same time. The ultimate winning combination!

Do this for each of your three liver-boosting ideas:

1. _____

2. _____

3. _____

Hormones

The collective term for all the glands that produce and secrete hormones is the 'endocrine system'. Hormones are chemical messengers created by the body; they transfer information from one set of cells to another to coordinate the functions of different parts of the body. Hormones regulate the body's growth and metabolism (all the physical and chemical processes of the body), as well as sexual development and function. Hormones are released into the bloodstream and may affect one or several organs throughout the body. In the case of weight loss, if even one hormone is out of balance, then others can be affected, restricting your body's ability to burn fat.

Once hormones have been produced by glands, they are released into the bloodstream as needed; they are a bit like letters or parcels that have been written and are waiting to be posted. These parcels are being sent all over your body 24/7, and determine your metabolic rate and to a large extent how your body functions.

Each hormone has a specific role. For example, insulin lowers blood sugar and converts excess glucose into fat, while glucagon increases blood sugar and promotes fat burning to provide energy in between meals. For a constant supply of energy without the highs and lows, these two hormones must work in balance. We will look at the vital role insulin plays in weight loss in more detail a little later on.

Just as a parcel can be sent recorded delivery, each hormonal message sent to a cell demands a receipt or a response. The cells have receivers, much like a letterbox, through which they receive the information. If the receiver is blocked it's like a letterbox being the wrong shape and the parcel cannot be delivered. There are times when you are producing the right hormone, but it is being blocked from doing its work. This is called a 'feedback system' and in this way information passes between the glands and the brain to decide how much of a particular hormone is needed; in a healthy body production and release of all hormones is balanced.

An example of when this system doesn't work is when chemicals that mimic hormones – such as pesticides – enter the bloodstream, or when hormones in the food chain are consumed, throwing our own hormone production out of balance by disrupting the feedback mechanism. One example of this is oestrogen. This is a female sex hormone that is involved in reproduction and also in fat storage. It is oestrogen that directs fat to be stored just under the belly button and on the hips and thighs; after menopause, when these levels drop, fat deposition changes and you often see older women with lovely slim legs and big round tummies. If you have elevated oestrogen levels, then you are in fat-storing mode (fat cells themselves produce oestrogen).

As well as your naturally produced oestrogen, you may be consuming oestrogen in your diet if you eat a lot of farmed meat because the hormone is often used in animal feed. Chickens fed on a diet high in growth hormones can grow rapidly and be big enough to slaughter in six weeks, instead of the 22 weeks it would take them to grow and develop naturally. Animal feeds that contain a cocktail of hormones to promote rapid growth are highly lucrative and widely used. It is no coincidence that, since hormones have started indirectly entering our food chain in this way, and the contraceptive pill has increased the amount of oestrogen in the water, the age of puberty has reduced. Men are also having more problems with fertility – and some even develop 'man boobs'.

Hormones not only control your appetite, the drive to eat and where fat is stored, but as you know from your own experience, they also affect your mood. We have already looked at the ability of serotonin to make us feel relaxed, less stressed and less prone to cravings. There's another hormone that makes us feel good. It's called oxytocin, and it's produced in the hypothalamus.

Oxytocin is often called the 'cuddle hormone' and Cupid's arrow is said to have been dipped in it! We release oxytocin when we feel love, trust and comfort, and it can be even more powerful than serotonin. If you need a lift, you can tap into the power of simply spending time with your family and friends, and of course your loved one. Even interacting with pets can release hormones that make us feel good; several studies have shown the therapeutic benefits of dog 'visitors' to long-term patients in hospitals and homes. When you are happy and contented, and not under stress, the drive to eat when you're not hungry disappears.

Insulin

Insulin is one of the better known hormones, and like all hormones it is essential for health. Simply put, one of insulin's main functions in the body is to control what goes into and out of cells, including glucose and fat. Insulin is largely responsible for maintaining optimal blood glucose levels, as a rise *or* a fall in blood glucose can have serious consequences for our health.

Glucose is the primary energy source in our bodies and *every* cell needs it. It makes sense therefore that we have the right amount circulating in our blood so it can be delivered to our cells. It is insulin's job to monitor and maintain blood glucose levels and respond to changing requirements. Clearly, the demand for fuel goes up when we are active, but glucose alone can't meet all our needs for energy because we just don't store enough of it (an average adult stores just over 2,000 calories as glucose). So when levels get low, we add fat to the mixture (we can store literally billions of calories of this!) to make up the deficit.

Think of a hybrid car. It is designed to run on two fuels – electricity (via a battery) and petrol (or diesel) from the storage tank. The amount of charge in the battery, and the power required by the engine at any given time, determine which fuel is used. When battery levels are fully charged and energy demand is low – for example when we are pottering around at low speed – no petrol is needed because the battery can meet all the demands for energy. However, on longer distances and at a higher speed, the battery charge drops quickly, so the car burns petrol as well as using the charge from the battery to make up the deficit.

In much the same way, the amount of glucose in your blood determines how much fat you burn in relation to the demands for energy. When glucose levels are high, and activity is low to moderate, little fat is needed, but when glucose levels are low and energy requirements go up, you need to add fat to the mixture to keep the supply constant. For effective fat burning and weight loss, then, you need a combination of glucose *and* fat (as you will see in chapter 10, which looks at exercise). While you can burn glucose without fat, *you cannot burn fat without glucose.*

If there's too much circulating glucose, you use this for energy instead of burning fat to bring blood glucose levels down naturally; insulin makes sure of this by blocking fat burning. Any excess glucose that can't be burnt as fuel is converted into fat. This process is initiated by insulin, so you can see what a vital role this hormone plays in weight loss!

Insulin Resistance

In a healthy person, the pancreas produces insulin. In someone with Type 1 diabetes, the pancreas cannot produce it, so it has to be injected. Years ago, people with this type of diabetes simply deteriorated and died. Today it is a manageable condition rather than a disease. In Type 2 diabetes the body does produce insulin but it is not usable – the cells cannot respond to it as they should. Medication is used to correct this, and diet and exercise also play a key role. In many cases Type 2 diabetes is reversible with a good regime.

In recent years a new condition that is also characterized by the body's inability to use insulin has been discovered. Similar in part to Type 2 diabetes, it is called insulin resistance, or IR. The condition is also the cause of Polycystic Ovary Syndrome, or PCOS (an imbalance of hormones that can cause serious health problems and infertility), because hyperinsulinemia (high insulin) has an impact on ovarian function. There is also a strong link between insulin and the adrenals (as you will see, many of the symptoms of imbalance are similar) as the whole endocrine system has to be in balance for optimum health.

The reality is that most people who are obese are probably insulin resistant. If you think about the word 'resistant', it gives you a clue as to what the condition actually means. Something is preventing something else from happening. Have you ever tried to unlock a door with a key that seems to fit into the lock, yet the mechanics aren't quite right and the key won't turn? That's exactly what happens with insulin resistance: the lock on the cell doesn't recognize insulin as the key and prevents it from working.

Remember the description earlier about the parcel being sent recorded delivery? Imagine it can't be delivered now because there's no one there to sign for it. When this happens in IR, blood sugar levels don't go down (as insulin is struggling to get it into cells), so the body produces more and more insulin to try and get the job done. It's a bit like shouting if someone can't hear you – if they are deaf, it doesn't matter how loud you shout, they won't hear. As a result of this increase in insulin production, fat burning is blocked.

Here are some of the non-medical symptoms of insulin resistance:

- Feeling tired even after a full night's sleep
- Inability to get to sleep, or waking in the early hours
- Giddiness when moving from a seated position to standing
- Stretch marks and brown pigments in the skin
- Unexplained fatigue
- Weight gain – especially in the mid-section
- Erratic or painful periods
- Inability to focus or concentrate
- Intestinal bloating and gas
- Tired after eating
- Difficulty losing weight
- Facial hair, or any excessive hair (in women)
- Mood swings
- Depression
- Excessive hunger and food cravings.

Medical symptoms include:

- High circulating insulin levels
- High blood glucose
- Increased blood triglycerides (fats)
- Increased blood pressure.

Although insulin resistance is a relatively 'new' condition, the association between a disorder of carbohydrate metabolism (balancing blood sugar) and the endocrine system (glands and hormones) was first described as early as 1921. Even today, many GPs are only just being informed of the significance of this condition, and as a result many people have to seek a private diagnosis because traditional glucose tolerance tests can't diagnose insulin resistance and the IR test is not available through many GPs. For more information on how to get tested privately visit www.medichecks.com. They will send a nurse out to collect your blood and give you a professional analysis and report as well as a telephone consultation when your results are ready.

Even if you are IR, the guidelines will be exactly the same as I'm giving you in this programme. This will become much clearer when you have read the exercise and nutrition sections (chapters 10 and 11) and have seen the simplicity of the colour code system in chapter 12. In addition to what you eat, *you must exercise* in order to change your hormonal production and balance. Sitting around and being inactive is a cause of fatness, not a cure. If you are IR and you do not address it, you are at increased risk of heart disease and other conditions.

In a normal, healthy body the natural production of insulin works very well on a simple 'feedback system' (messages being sent recorded delivery and being signed for): we eat, blood sugar goes up, and the right amount of insulin is released to put the glucose into the cells that need it. While glucose levels are high, insulin stops fat from being used for energy as it's simply not needed. When the circulating glucose levels drop, and energy requirements are not being met, then fat is released to make up the difference.

An insulin resistant body may have an insulin response 5–10 times greater than a healthy body. This explains why some people can eat the same foods as others and not gain fat. Some of this may be genetic, but these genes can be 'turned off' and hormones up-regulated or down-regulated depending on your lifestyle. So, the good news is, with the right nutrition, and regular exercise to improve your body's composition and reduce the ratio of fat to muscle (lean body mass – or LBM), you can restore the balance. It won't happen overnight though – it will take time to get your body into the healthy state you desire and become a fat burner.

Make it a priority to manage your blood sugar, because it is high blood sugar (or glucose) that triggers the extra insulin release and the subsequent increase in fat storing. If you focus on preventing high blood glucose, rather than on losing weight at any cost, the fat and the inches will come off automatically. You will also feel so much better!

A Personal Story About Insulin Resistance

I was lucky to meet Professor Nadir Farid, a brilliant endocrinologist whose pioneering work on insulin resistance helped my daughter Emilie get the diagnosis she needed after several years of feeling unwell and suffering some of the extremely unpleasant symptoms of IR and PCOS, and struggling with her weight. When Emilie was 16 (she's now 21), we were told that everything she was going through was normal for her age. But I knew this was not the case, and I was determined to find a way to help her.

I knew in my heart, and through my training, that nutrition and exercise were key, but I didn't know exactly what the problem was. After watching Professor Farid speak at a seminar, I immediately recognized the symptoms of IR in Emilie. I just sat and cried, partly with relief because I'd finally found some answers, and partly with concern for her future. I spoke to Professor Farid after the seminar and he immediately agreed to see Emilie. Thanks to him, she now has a clear strategy to manage her condition and some serious health consequences have been avoided before they fully began. With a Type 1 diabetic grandmother (insulin dependent), Emilie was genetically predisposed to problems, but now, with the right nutrition and exercise, she is likely to avoid becoming diabetic. I have no doubt that she would now be in a very different place, health-wise, if I hadn't attended the seminar that day.

More About Glucose

You may have heard athletes use the term 'hitting the wall'. This refers to the point in extreme exercise when there is no more glucose left in the body. We have a 'survival mechanism' to deal with this – it's a special facility that is designed to protect us in times of famine. However, as you will see, when we diet it's easy to trick the body into using this mechanism. When blood glucose is getting low, we use more and more fat mixed with the glucose to make it last longer; you could say fat dilutes the glucose to keep the energy supply going, but eventually, with extreme exercise such as marathon running, glucose runs out.

When this happens we literally cannibalize our own muscle tissue to release the tiny glucose strands within the muscle to provide us (primarily our brains) with the energy we need to function. This state is called 'ketosis'. This was a very useful mechanism for our hunter-gatherer ancestors, who had times of famine and had to go hunting all day to chase and catch their food. Today, ketosis can be initiated in exactly the same way, simply by eating a high-protein, low-carb diet.

You will learn more about this in later chapters, but just think about that and let me repeat it again because it is hugely important:

When we run out of glucose, we cannibalize our muscle tissue (lean body mass, or LBM) to provide the brain with the glucose it needs. This is significant because the only place in our body that burns fat is muscle (LBM). When you cannibalize LBM, you are reducing your ability to burn fat.

Dr Atkins had it half right when he 'created' the high-protein diet, but sadly his approach (and those of the others who jumped on the same lucrative bandwagon) failed to appreciate the overall consequence on body composition, and overall health. His principle was simple: if insulin causes fat storage and blocks fat burning, then let's create a system to prevent insulin from being produced. Then we can't get fat! Sounds too good to be true, eh? It is. We *need* insulin, and when we deliberately suppress insulin production it triggers a series of chain reactions that lead to long-term health problems, some of which can be fatal. This is why we give diabetics insulin – without it we die!

The ketones (produced when we are in ketosis) are a by-product of fat metabolism and are used for energy when circulating glucose is dangerously low. Your brain (which has a dominant need for glucose) does not function well on ketones and it is certainly *not* a desirable condition. If your GP tests your urine and detects ketones, you have been officially diagnosed with a metabolic dysfunction. Yet for some reason in the high-protein community, this dysfunction is seen as a success – even desirable! You are told to go to the chemist to buy a kit to measure your own urine so you can make sure you *are* in ketosis!

Millions of people, all chasing the promise of weight loss, flocked like lambs to the slaughter to follow this advice. That's bloody scary! I have no doubt that Dr Atkins was well intentioned, but the long-term effects of a high-protein diet include kidney failure, heart disease and osteoporosis, to name but a few. Several deaths have been attributed to this regime, too – well, that's certainly one way to lose weight! The answer is to manage our insulin levels so we produce enough to maintain normal healthy function, but avoid the overproduction, or 'spiking', that is caused by eating foods that contain too much glucose.

This is one of the key components in the colour code system in chapter 12 – you eat foods that release their glucose slowly, so you don't get the insulin 'spikes' that cause weight gain. You will see when you follow the colour code guidelines how simple this can be. This chapter is just to give you an understanding of how and why the colour code system works so well. My own studies have shown that when you understand the principles behind any system you are following, and you have confidence in it, it's easier for your unconscious mind to accept all the new things you are learning, and you can easily adapt your behaviours to make the changes you need to make.

So, now you understand how balancing your hormones is crucial for weight loss – both physiologically and emotionally. Let's now have a look at some specific glands and how you can boost your fat-burning potential naturally.

The Adrenals

The adrenal glands sit at the top of the kidneys and are largely responsible for managing your body's stress levels. When you are under stress, you produce a different set of hormones than you do when you are relaxed and peaceful. Because your energy requirements are different when you are stressed, this directly affects fat storage. When your adrenals are stressed, you store more fat – typically around the mid-section – you may also notice some facial hair, a bloated face and puffy eyes.

Your adrenals control your sleep patterns via circadian rhythms so when they are stressed you don't achieve peaceful, restful sleep and find you are tired all day. Despite being 'exhausted' by the time you go to bed, you can't sleep, or you wake up at 2 a.m. for no apparent reason and can't get back to sleep for ages. You may also notice that you get out of breath easily and are more prone to stress – little things make you anxious, you develop a very short fuse and worry a lot. You may get very thirsty but despite consuming lots of fluids, the reduced sodium levels associated with this condition make it difficult for water to be absorbed into the cells, so you remain dehydrated. Some of the body's serotonin is produced by the adrenals and as you now know, this can lead to an increase in cravings.

Here are some guidelines for keeping your adrenals healthy. Specific foods that boost adrenal function are listed in chapter 12.

- **Avoid high-sugar foods.**
- **Avoid refined foods,** even if they contain no visible added sugar.
- **Eat slow-releasing foods** (see chapter 12 for a list of these).
- **Avoid too much caffeine.**
- **Avoid getting really hungry.**
- **Eat healthy, good-quality snacks,** such as fruit and nuts.
- **Eat high-quality proteins** like fish (wild or organic); organic chicken; organic beans and lentils; lean, lightly cooked red meat (rare meat is easier to digest); and fresh, raw nuts.
- **Eat lots of raw and lightly cooked vegetables** (including salads).
- **Avoid artificial sweeteners.**
- **Reduce stress levels.**

The Thyroid

This is the gland that regulates your body's metabolism. In other words, it controls the speed at which you burn fuel. The thyroid works a bit like the accelerator in a car – you can either go faster or slower depending on the environment. If you go faster, you burn more fuel, if you go slower you conserve fuel. The environment in this case is determined by your hormones – how much (and what) you are eating, how active you are, and your overall health. The thyroid also determines your body temperature, just like a thermostat.

The thyroid is situated in the throat and, if it is dysfunctional, can appear quite large. An overactive thyroid means your metabolic rate is too high. Extreme weight loss occurs, you become irrational, and eye sockets can contract, giving the appearance of protruding eye balls. An underactive thyroid means the reverse – sufferers become sluggish, mentally and physically fatigued, and gain weight that is difficult to shift. This weight tends to be general and not as site-specific as when your liver is dysfunctional (pot belly) or your adrenals are stressed (tummy).

There is a strong link between your thyroid gland and your ovaries, which produce oestrogen. This is especially relevant after menopause, a time when a lot of women gain weight. The majority of thyroid function occurs through the liver, where thyroid hormones are broken down, so a healthy liver is vital. Exercise can also stimulate thyroid function, and there's more about this a little later in the book.

To boost thyroid function you need to combine regular exercise with a nutrient-rich diet. Iodine is the key nutrient required for thyroid function and a deficiency in it will lead to an underactive thyroid.

Here are some foods that are rich in iodine:

- **Sea vegetables** (i.e. kelp)
- **Yoghurt**
- **Cow's milk** (stick to organic if possible)
- **Eggs** (preferably organic)
- **Strawberries**
- **Mozzarella cheese**
- **Fish and shellfish.**

Exercise
· · · · · · · ·

Think about and then list three things you can do every day that will increase your thyroid function and therefore your ability to burn fat. Then read them out loud, as you did for the two exercises above.

1. _____

2. _____

3. _____

Stress

De-stressing is an undervalued component of weight loss. I've had clients take up yoga and think that it must somehow be burning more calories than aerobics because they start to lose weight despite having been previously 'stuck'! The reality is this: when you are stressed you release cortisol, which blocks the fat-burning process. If you blast away like a bat out of hell on the treadmill after a hard day at the office you put your body under a different kind of stress. Even if you enjoy it, it's still a form of stress and can reduce the amount of fat you can burn after exercise.

I'm not suggesting that you shouldn't do aerobic exercise – far from it. You *should* do aerobic exercise and resistance training to maximize fat burning! But you must also find a way of exercising, or some other technique, such as meditation, that relaxes you and doesn't over-stress your body. It may be that you do the aerobics class, but then finish with some yoga or meditation to relax and balance your hormones.

Believe me, when you do this you'll not only burn more fat after your exercise, you'll sleep better and your body will be able to complete the valuable process of growth and repair undisturbed by stress hormones. Learning to meditate, and doing it for just 10 minutes before you go to sleep, can be a great way to de-stress and balance your hormones for the body's night-time processes. Some of the growth hormones responsible for fat burning are produced by your body at night, when you are in restful sleep. If you don't achieve restful sleep, you produce very few of these hormones and long-term fat metabolism is impaired. You can download a free audio relaxation guide at www.powertochange. me.uk (click on the *Think More, Eat Less* link and use the password 'Positive Attitude').

Exercise
. . . .

Think about and then write down three things you can do every day that will reduce your stress levels and therefore increase your ability to burn fat. You could try some of the psychological exercises from earlier in the book. Use the technique of repeating them out loud described earlier. Do it – it's important. If you are too lazy to do this, then why are you reading this book!? Just do it!

1. _____

2. _____

3. _____

Mabel's Journal

Bloody hell. This chapter was such an eye-opener for me! I can't believe how amazing the human body is. At school, biology seemed to pass me by, but I found this fascinating, and a little scary, but in a good way, because instead of blaming being fat on my hormones, I realize to my surprise that I can actually control them – without taking pills! This really is a bit of a revelation. I mean, everyone should know this stuff!

I've read through each bit of this chapter with great interest, trying to see which body systems relate the most to me. I could see that actually ALL of them need some TLC. I think I need to look after my liver much more carefully, and certainly the symptoms of insulin resistance describe me to a T. Not sure if I am scared or relieved??

Can't imagine how Janet felt when she discovered her daughter had it as early as a teenager, but actually my symptoms and weight gain all started about that time too.

My doctor has been telling me for years that if I don't lose weight I'll probably become diabetic, but it was as if I didn't really hear it or apply it to me – until now! This is a BIG wake up call. I understand now why I suffered from constant backache when I was on the high-protein diet. My poor kidneys were trying to tell me something. I should have guessed, because within a week of stopping it, the backache went. Why was I so gullible? At least now I know exactly what my body needs and I won't be seduced by any fad diet EVER AGAIN! Interesting to see what the 'diet' in this book will be? I've kind of worked it out already after reading this chapter, but am intrigued about the colour code system. Hope it's not complicated, because I REALLY want to sort my body out once and for all.

When I went for my walk tonight, I actually jogged for over five minutes and went a bit further than usual. The thought of exercise helping to balance my hormone levels inspired me even more. It was a bit grey and murky and looked like rain – any other time I would have taken one look out the window and not bothered! But I want to have happy hormones every day, not just on sunny days, so I got off my arse and did it! Going to do the relaxation meditation from the website tonight, and burn fat while I sleep! Now there's a concept I really like!!

Chapter 10

FAT CELLS OR FLAT CELLS?

Your fat cells – those things that store your fat and make you look flabby – are actually tiny, minute in fact. The size of a typical fat cell in an adult of a 'healthy weight' is about 0.6 micrograms (a microgram is one millionth of a gram, so fats cells are pretty small). However, they can expand. To what size depends on the individual, but it's estimated the maximum expansion is 0.9 micrograms. When they are full, fat cells have the ability to replicate, as happens in obese individuals.

The good news is that when they are empty, the minute size of fat cells means we don't look fat and flabby anymore! Some scientists now view fat cells as part of the endocrine system, because they aren't as dormant as was once thought – they actually produce oestrogen and other chemical messages. If protein is the building block of muscles, fat is the building blob of fat!

How To Shrink Your Fat Cells

I am going to keep this part quite brief. You are smart and you already know most of the key points I'm going to teach you now. But the foremost among them is this: *get moving*! If you want to burn fat you *must* move your body. I told you earlier that the only place your body burns fat is in your muscles, so you *must* move and strengthen your muscles. Otherwise it would be like having a car in the garage that burns fat instead of petrol. If you never take it out of the garage, or only do short journeys, it burns very little fat, despite its potential!

Essentially, there are two types of exercise – aerobic and anaerobic. Aerobic simply means 'with oxygen'. Aerobic is the only system that actually burns fat. Three things need to combine to produce energy 'aerobically' – fat, oxygen and glucose. Fat cannot be burnt on its own though. It's a shame really, otherwise you could just get up in the morning, go for a 10-hour walk and come home at the end of the day a stone lighter! Sadly, our bodies don't work like that. They simply can't burn fat without oxygen and glucose. It's a simple law of physics. In the same way you can't light a fire without the presence of oxygen, within your cells you can't burn fat without oxygen and glucose. All three must be present for the combustion of the fat to take place.

Your aerobic capacity is entirely dependent on the ability of your cardiovascular system to pump oxygen (which is carried in red blood cells) around the body. If you have a weak heart and circulation system, your ability to exercise is restricted because you can't get the oxygen you need delivered to your muscles to move them. As you know from the previous chapter, glucose (from carbohydrate) is used *by every cell, all the time.* It is the primary source of energy for everyday functions. Your brain, in particular, has a dominant need for glucose, and if levels within your body drop too low, you have a special in-built survival mechanism that literally breaks down your muscle tissue and converts it into glucose (producing ketones) to meet the brain's need for fuel. Critically, you do *not* need oxygen or anything else to burn glucose for energy.

Many diets (high-protein, low-carb based diets in particular) use this theory to achieve weight loss, i.e. restricting glucose supply so that instead you use fat to meet your energy needs. As another function of glucose is to enable us to store water within our cells, the combined fluid and muscle loss can be quite drastic on the scales, but in reality you end up with a higher percentage of body fat even though you weigh less. You are lighter, but flabbier. As I explained in the last chapter, when glucose levels drop too low you compensate by metabolizing your own muscle, or LBM, which is the key factor in determining how many calories you are able to burn every day.

When you go back to 'normal' eating, you cannot physically burn as many calories as you did before because your LBM determines your metabolic rate – less LBM means a lower metabolic rate, so you not only regain any weight lost (usually as more fat), but gain extra fat as well. In this way it's very easy to use what is essentially a survival mechanism to diet yourself fat. Does this sound familiar? The answer is not to have so much glucose that you don't need to burn fat, but not too little that you need to cannibalize your muscle tissue to make up the deficit. It's all about balance.

A diet too high in protein and too low in carbs can also disrupt the body's natural balance, including its pH levels, which can lead to osteoporosis, kidney damage, heart disease and many other serious health consequences. Protein is important, essential in fact, but in the right quantities.

Getting the balance of nutrients right is what forms the basis of the colour code system you will learn in chapter 12, and you can be confident that all the calculations have been done for you. If you choose the right number of foods from the right colour groups, you will be nourishing your body, helping to balance your hormones, and enhancing your fat-burning capabilities.

Burning Fat

So, you now know that the key to effective fat burning is to ensure you have the right amount of glucose in your bloodstream to meet your body's needs, so that when challenged with activity or movement, it has to dip into your fat stores, which it then blends with the glucose and burns using oxygen. Every time you move your muscles, you are burning some fat; you are also burning some fat at rest, and even at night. When you sleep restfully, the hormones that promote fat burning are stimulated – the amount you burn is dependent on what you have eaten, how active you've been, your hormone levels and the amount of LBM you have.

Every time you exercise, the hormones and enzymes that release and burn fat become more efficient. The growth and repair of your muscle tissue – which occurs overnight during restful sleep – builds healthier, stronger muscles – increasing your lean body mass (LBM). This enables you to burn more fat every day, even when you are not exercising.

The graphic below shows how all these things combine to make you efficient at burning fat.

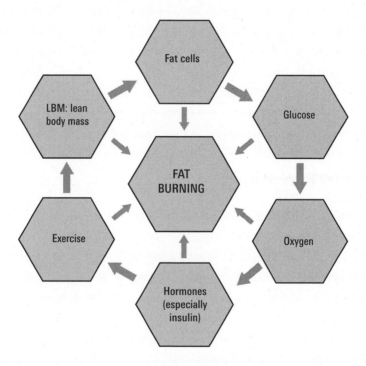

Anaerobic means 'without oxygen'. Remember, you can burn glucose on its own without fat or oxygen (but not the other way around), and you do this in all cells except muscle cells, which use fat and oxygen as well as glucose. When you are weight training you are working anaerobically: you are loading one specific muscle group for a very short period of time. Let's say you are doing a leg press exercise in the gym. The exercise set may be over in less than a minute, so your body doesn't have time to send a message out to your fat cells, asking them to release the fat into your bloodstream and then direct it through the circulation system to your thigh muscles to mix with glucose and oxygen.

However, if you were to use your thigh muscles for power walking or cycling, then the workload would be much lower. After all, you can walk for a lot longer than you can do a heavy leg press, so you are much more likely to keep the activity going for longer. Now your body does have time to liberate fat from the cells, circulate it and get it to the working muscles on a constant basis.

Which Exercise Is Best?

In reality, we are always using a combination of both aerobic and anaerobic 'systems'. Humans are aerobic creatures – we cannot survive without oxygen – but as you learnt in the section on insulin, we also have the ability to switch energy systems according to the demands on our body and which fuel supplies we have available. The difference is not dissimilar to that of comparing electricity with gas: if you walk into a cold room and you want instant energy, you put on an electric fan heater; if you want longer-term heat then you put on the central heating, which, although takes longer to work, is very efficient and can last for hours. Electricity is like using glucose alone – it's immediately available, whereas central heating is like mixing glucose with oxygen and fat – it takes longer to get going because it relies on a circulation system to be delivered, just like your radiators need hot water to be pumped from the boiler.

An aerobic activity such as power walking, jogging or cycling will become anaerobic as you get more tired and your heart has to work harder to supply the oxygen. At the beginning of a 30-minute workout, assuming you have warmed up correctly and raised your heart rate gradually, you will be working mainly aerobically. After about 15 minutes, if you are beginning to feel a little more challenged, the ratio will change slightly – you will be using less fat and oxygen as your circulation is struggling to keep up delivery, and relying more on glucose. If by the end of 30 minutes you are wiped out, you will be in your anaerobic zone (relying almost totally on glucose), which you can't sustain for more than a few minutes. This is when athletes 'hit the wall'. In a fit individual this takes a marathon to reach, but in a very unfit individual it can be reached after as little as a few minutes of activity.

In terms of burning fat, we have established that you burn fat when you work aerobically, *but* there is also an energy cost *after* you've finished exercising that also burns fat, and this is determined by the intensity of the workout. In simple terms, the harder you work out during your exercise session, the more fat you burn afterwards. So, comparing activities and how much fat they burn when you do them can be very misleading.

There are four key components to an effective exercise regime, and these are shown in the graphic below.

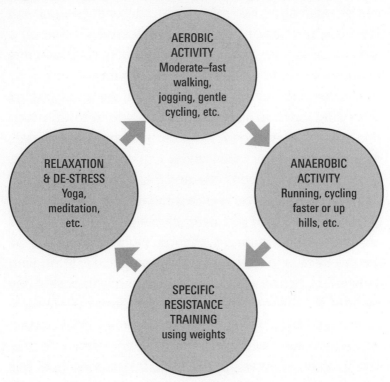

Anaerobic exercise in particular has been shown to be beneficial for boosting thyroid function – specifically when working at 70 per cent or above of your maximum heart rate. So short bursts of intense activity, such as running and cycling (assuming you are fit enough) are beneficial as part of your overall exercise regime. This is something you can work up to gradually if your fitness levels are currently low. A mixture of high and low intensity exercise on different days will yield the best results.

Resistance training, i.e. with weights, will increase your metabolic rate so you burn more calories, even when you are not exercising. Resistance training increases your lean body mass (LBM), which is made up primarily of muscle. Always remember this: the *only* cells in your body that can burn fat are your muscle cells, so if you increase the strength and efficiency of your muscles (your LBM), your ability to burn fat increases, even when you are not exercising. This is so important it is worth repeating: *only muscles burn fat*!

Any exercise regime designed to promote fat loss *must* include some form of resistance exercise that will replace some of the natural muscle wastage that comes with age and inactivity. Every pound of muscle burns 40 calories per day at rest, so if you can increase your muscle density, your everyday fat-burning potential is drastically increased. This is why on some programmes there is a visible change in body composition – your clothes become looser and you look and feel better, but there is negligible weight loss on the scales. This does level out after a while, but as long as you are losing inches, and starting to look and feel better, don't worry if you are not losing as much weight as you think you should be. You are changing your body composition and that will lead to a long-term loss of fat.

Taking It Slowly

One client once told me she had been exercising regularly, had been 'really good' with her food, felt her clothes were getting looser, but when she went for her weekly weigh-in at her slimming club she was 'told off' for only losing half a pound. She immediately went home, ate six slices of toast and gave up. Three years later, and now two stone heavier, she came to see me. This happens all the time and it's purely down to not understanding how the body works and responds to change. Always remember the Three Little Pigs: the quickest way is not the best way and what looks good from the outside often doesn't last. If you are losing inches, then you are losing fat weight.

The primary goal is to get fit and healthy, so your hormones can function properly to allow you to burn fat. Depending on your start point – how out-of-balance your system is – it may take a few weeks for this to correct before you start to see significant weight loss. Be patient though, and focus on balancing your system first – when you do this, the weight will come off naturally.

One final point about exercise. For as many years as I can remember, the question I'm asked most about exercise is: 'Which is the best exercise for weight loss?' Having given you the technical information above, you now know the academic answer to that, but in reality the correct answer is: 'The exercise you most enjoy doing', because that's the only one you are likely to stick to.

When I'm asked, 'How hard should I work?' my answer is, 'As hard as you can for as long as you can, and as often as you can – depending on your fitness level'. That way you maximize the calories you burn when you work out, but also increase your metabolic rate on the days you are not working out. Keep in mind that relaxation and de-stressing should also make up part of your regime.

Ideally, you will combine a mixture of different activities so you can work aerobically and also build LBM. Bear in mind when designing your activity or exercise regime that it has to be something you *enjoy*. Even a game of badminton twice a week or a Zumba class will burn calories and get you moving. So the bottom line is this: just do something!

Exercise

Write down three things you can do regularly that will increase your body's ability to burn fat, then say each one out loud with emotion:

1. _____

   _____

2. _____

   _____

3. _____

   _____

Mabel's Journal

After reading this chapter yesterday I went to the sports centre gym on the way home and signed up. I am DEFINITELY going to increase my LBM (now I know what it is!!). Got my induction tomorrow, going for a walk today and determined to jog a bit further.

~~~~~~~~~~

Well, my body must be wondering what's happened to it over the last 24 hours! Yesterday I managed to jog for almost 10 minutes of my 20-minute 'walk', and today I was shown how to use the resistance equipment at the gym. My trainer must have wondered what was going on when this overweight woman walked up to him and told him exactly what she wanted to do. I bet he thought, 'How can she know so much and yet be so fat!' Well not for much longer!!! I didn't overdo it, but my body is really feeling it today. It doesn't hurt, but I definitely reached parts of my body that thought they'd been relieved of duty!!!

My goal is to go to the gym at least once a week and to carry on my walking/jogging three times. On the day I go to the gym I could do my aerobic bit on the treadmill there, and when the weather gets a bit colder I'll have to go there all the time because I'm definitely not stopping now. Well on my way to being able to run for 30 minutes by Christmas because it's only April! Might even try a Zumba class if I'm feeling brave!

Going to do the relaxation audio again now. Have downloaded it on to my iPod. Gonna burn more fat while I sleep :o)

Chapter 11

FOOD MATTERS

Earlier in the book I told you how, when I was researching my Master's degree dissertation, I wanted to show that if people record what they eat, they automatically choose healthier foods, and as a result, lose more weight. My results did show that, but I also found an unexpected benefit of teaching people about how to eat well – during the six weeks of the nutrition course that I ran prior to the actual study, the average weight loss was greater than in the 10 weeks that followed. Despite the fact that I'd asked my volunteers not to change what they ate until the study began, almost all of them made small changes that had a significant impact on their weight. Many of them lost a dress size without even consciously trying! It didn't help my study at the time, but it did teach me a valuable lesson that I have used to help many people since: Knowledge Is Power.

Having proven that food recording is a helpful tool for achieving weight loss, I also realized that for most people, writing down everything you eat is a real pain. I wanted to create a system that made food recording simple, so I separated the main food groups into different colours, and simply asked people to make a note of how many portions of each colour they ate. Of course, I had to give them guidelines to follow about many portions of each colour would be best. After two years of trialling different combinations and colours, and analyzing numerous diets, I created the colour code system that you see in the next chapter. Since then I've continued to refine and improve it, and the system I'm bringing you now is, I believe, the very best way to follow a well-balanced 'diet', without actually dieting.

What Makes A Good 'Diet'?

Before we get into the colour code system itself, let me give you an overview of it, and teach you a few key facts about nutrients – how they are digested and what your body needs nutritionally to be healthy *and* to burn fat.

The word 'diet' simply means what you eat – or scientifically speaking, 'your energy intake' or EI. So in truth, we are *all* on a diet. It's the slimming diet mentality that's the problem, though, because it involves deprivation or avoidance – often of valuable nutrients – for the sole purpose of losing weight and with little or no regard for the long-term impact on our health. All that stops now!

It's currently very fashionable to base 'diets' on what our ancestors ate – specifically cavemen, who were hunter-gatherers. I find the fixation with eating the same as cavemen somewhat bemusing, because cavemen had a significantly shorter lifespan than we do. They were also probably extremely hungry a lot of the time, and had to eat what was available rather than choose their foods based on what tasted, smelt or looked good. There are, of course, elements of this 'diet' that are good, but not the complete concept. The reason cavemen were slim was due as much to the fact that they were highly active physically, and that their diets contained no high-fat, high-sugar foods, or indeed any excess of food. I really enjoy my food, so this sort of restrictive regime doesn't appeal to me one bit!

However, it is clear that when high-sugar, high-fat foods are unavailable, our diets are automatically much healthier. One example of this was seen in the period during and immediately after World War II, when rationing was in force. Meat was in short supply and people had to rely a lot more on homegrown vegetables. There are elements of this postwar 'deprivation' that would benefit us today. Engine fuel was also rationed, so although people didn't have to chase their dinners, they did have to walk everywhere instead of taking the car. It is no coincidence that the population at this time was slimmer and the incidence of heart disease was much lower.

The reality is that there are some good elements to most diets – it's just that they are so often taken to extremes. The high-protein diet, for example, was initially based on some sound concepts, but these were made so extreme that they became potentially very harmful to health if sustained. Refined foods such as bread, rice or pasta are not allowed on the high-protein diet and it's recommended that lots of lean meat and fish be consumed. These elements of the diet are sound up to a point, but others – such as consuming little or no fruit – should be ignored. Doing that would be to deny your body the valuable antioxidant (cancer-preventive) nutrients that it simply must have, as well as the many phytochemicals and fibre these foods contain. More about this in the section on carbohydrates.

There seems to be a fixation with coming up with faddy, fashionable diets in which some obvious concepts are ignored for fear of being boring, or not 'sexy' enough to market. I will not bow to that pressure! Instead, I will give you the information you need, and then show you how to adapt the colour code system to make it work for you. One thing's for sure, no more faddy dieting (and I'll leave the 'sexy' bit to you!!)

You *can* calculate approximately how many calories you need to consume on a daily basis, but unless you are actually going to count *every* calorie you eat, there's little point. In the colour code system, if you stick to the guidelines and the portion sizes, you will probably be eating around 1,800 calories per day. If you are active, this is enough to lose weight and satisfy you at the same time. You may not even be able to eat this amount! However, you should *never* go below 1,500 calories per day, as this can result in a drop in your metabolic rate and reduce your capacity to burn fat.

Here in the Western world, our lifestyles have become increasingly sedentary, and this has impacted greatly on how much we need to eat. Our parents and grandparents were by necessity much more active than we are today. We actually need 30–50 per cent less energy than they did. This means that if we eat like they did, we'll get fat, and surprise surprise, we eat *even more* than they did, so we've got *really* fat!

The Three Key Nutrients

Fats, carbohydrates and protein are the three main nutrients (excluding water) that your body needs to function. They work together to provide energy and on-going growth and repair. When eaten in the right amounts, and from the right sources, they provide us with protection from disease, slow down the ageing process, and give us vitality and longevity.

The amount of each nutrient that you need as an individual varies and is determined largely by your activity levels and your age. For example, athletes and more active people need more carbohydrates than sedentary people because they have a higher energy requirement – also weight loss is not an issue for them as most of the glucose they ingest is used up quickly and they don't have to worry about the fat-storing effects of high blood sugar.

There is no set figure for the exact amount or percentage of each nutrient you should have in your diet, and two individuals may function better on slightly different amounts, depending on various factors, but the graphic below gives you a general guideline:

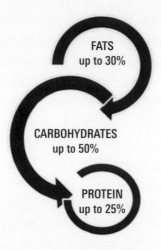

FATS
up to 30%

CARBOHYDRATES
up to 50%

PROTEIN
up to 25%

Fats should make up approximately 30 per cent of your diet. That does not mean that this percentage of your diet should be fish and chips, Chinese takeaways and ice-cream, though! There are two types of fat:

1. **Saturated Fatty Acids (SFAs)** – solid at body temperature (37°C / 98°F).

2. **Unsaturated Fatty Acids (UFAs)** – essential fatty acids or EFAs – liquid at body temperature.

Saturated Fatty Acids

SFAs are found in meat and animal products, including dairy. Chocolate is also a major source, and despite claims for its antioxidant properties, should be eaten in extreme moderation. An average bar of milk chocolate has approximately 9.1 grams of saturated fatty acids, which is 46 per cent of the RDA (Recommended Daily Allowance). Pure cocoa powder, on the other hand, has hardly any at all – less than 1 per cent. It's a good substitute for chocolate in baking, if you want to get the chocolate taste without the fat. Other animal products that are high in saturated fatty acids include processed meats such as pâté, which is also combined with butter and in most cases cream, making it a very high-calorie food. Hard cheese and butter are also full of SFAs. The only two saturated fatty acids that do not come from animal sources are coconut oil and palm oil.

If you want to consume the maximum amount of SFAs in one meal, then a lamb korma or pasanda would be about as high as you can get – especially if you have it with a naan bread, because that is also very high on the glycemic index or GI (see p.187). That meal contains more than 500 calories and would also be converted to fat; throw in a pint of beer or some wine and it would be difficult to find a more fat-storing meal! A much healthier Indian meal would be chicken tikka or tandoori, with a vegetable curry side dish and a small portion of basmati rice or a chapatti (not both!). With Chinese food, so much of it is fried that it's easy to consume lots of fatty and high GI foods. A good option there would be to have steamed fish with vegetables, and a small amount of boiled or steamed rice. If you stop yourself going to these kinds of restaurants you may feel like a bit of a pariah, socially. I love going for an Indian meal or getting a takeaway sometimes, but those are the type of dishes I choose.

In the first section of the book, you learnt about how your brain works and how important positive associations and emotions are, so it's *vital* that you learn to adapt the things you enjoy so you don't feel like you are on a diet. If you stop everything you like overnight, you are less likely to stick to the programme. In fact, I can almost guarantee you won't. Most meals, including trips to restaurants, can be managed with some careful choices and you won't have to drastically change your lifestyle.

SFAs – Friend Or Foe?

Some saturated fatty acids in the diet is acceptable; in fact if you are a meat eater, or enjoy hard cheese, then it's impossible not to get some. However, in the Western world most people consume far too many SFAs and not enough unsaturated fatty acids (UFAs), which has a huge and negative impact on our health. UFAs, and in particular the essential fatty acids omega-3 and omega-6, provide the structure for all cell membranes and are vital for good health. An excess of SFAs however, gets deposited in our fat stores and increases our risk of a whole range of diseases including heart disease, diabetes, stroke and cancer. Too much saturated fat is a killer. It looks bad from the outside and its effects are even worse on the inside.

Remember this: if a fat solidifies at room temperature (i.e. once it's out of the oven and cooled), it will solidify *inside* your body once digested. That's what makes it a saturated fatty acid. Think what your roasting tray looks like after you've cooked a joint of beef or lamb – there will be a sticky, white layer of fat in the bottom when it cools and that's exactly what will be happening inside your body when you've eaten it. The saturated fatty acids in meat have been stored there by the animal for the same reasons you store SFAs – for energy. So when you eat a lot of meat, it's not even *your* fat that's making you fat, you are getting 'ready-made' fat from the animal, who has done all the conversion for you! Fat has a calorific value of 9 calories per gram.

I don't need to tell you which fatty foods not to eat – you are too smart for that, am I right? If I have to cover the next few pages with a list of crisps, chips, chocolates, cakes etc., then you are in serious denial. What I may need to tell you about is the fats that you *do* need to eat: the fats that improve your health by helping to balance your hormones and also aid your metabolism, therefore helping you to lose weight.

Unsaturated Fatty Acids

The key difference between the two types of fat is that unsaturated fatty acids (UFAs) are liquid at room temperature, and therefore within the body. This liquidity means they can be used for things like cell membranes – in fact every cell in your body has a membrane made of UFAs. However, the fact they are so delicate that they can be used in this way also makes them fragile, and exposure to heat, light or even oxygen reduces or eliminates their nutritional qualities. This is why you pay so much more for extra virgin cold-pressed olive oil – it has been extracted from the olive in a cold, darkened room to preserve its quality. Good quality oils like this always come in darker bottles to protect them further from the light and should be stored in a cool, dark place. When it comes to cooking, use them for dressings but not for frying because that just destroys their natural qualities. Do add a few drops of extra-virgin oil to your roast potatoes or stir-fry *after* you've cooked them in regular or 'light' olive oil though, as this gives them extra flavour.

While we need some SFAs for insulation and for energy, we don't need much. It's an area of controversy among nutritionists but a guideline would be to eat a ratio of two or three UFAs to one SFA. Unsaturated fatty acids can be broken down further into monounsaturated fatty acids (MUFAs) and polyunsaturated fatty acids (PUFAs); these are also called essential fatty acids. We don't need to go into great detail here, but the difference between these is in the length of the carbon chain and how valuable and usable each is within the body. For our purposes we just need to know that you need *both*. You can see the foods that contain these different types of fat in the diagram opposite:

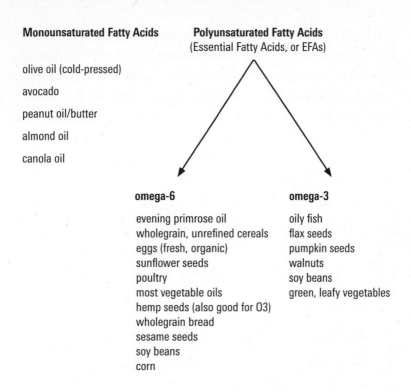

Monounsaturated Fatty Acids

olive oil (cold-pressed)

avocado

peanut oil/butter

almond oil

canola oil

Polyunsaturated Fatty Acids
(Essential Fatty Acids, or EFAs)

omega-6

evening primrose oil
wholegrain, unrefined cereals
eggs (fresh, organic)
sunflower seeds
poultry
most vegetable oils
hemp seeds (also good for O3)
wholegrain bread
sesame seeds
soy beans
corn

omega-3

oily fish
flax seeds
pumpkin seeds
walnuts
soy beans
green, leafy vegetables

The unsaturated fatty acids in food are more easily absorbed than those found in supplements, so although supplements can be useful, they are not intended to be replacements for UFAs in the diet. If you want to be healthy and slim, you must look at your diet and make sure you are taking in the right materials to carry out the job of making you slim! One of the easiest ways to get a good balance of omega-6 and omega-3 is to crush some fresh seeds every morning and sprinkle them on cereal just before eating; or at some other time in the day, toss them in a salad. An ideal blend would be flax and pumpkin (omega-3), with sesame and sunflower (omega-6). Because it's easier to consume omega-6 in the diet, use twice as much flax and pumpkin. Alternatively, you can grind some hemp seeds – these already contain a good balance of both essential fatty acids. Hemp seeds are from the marijuana plant, but the seeds do not make you high and can be sold legally in a health food shop!

If You're Not Getting Enough

The benefits of unsaturated fats, and in particular omega-6 and omega-3 are infinite in terms of your health. Rather than explain in detail what these essential fatty acids do, here's a list of some of the many symptoms of a deficiency in them:

- **Skin problems – especially dry skin conditions such as eczema**
- **Hair loss**
- **Liver degeneration**
- **Kidney degeneration**
- **Gland malfunction**
- **Susceptibility to infection**
- **Failure to heal**
- **Arthritis and other inflammatory conditions**
- **Heart and circulation problems**
- **Behavioural disturbances**
- **Growth retardation**
- **Impaired vision**
- **Tingling sensations in arms and legs**
- **Loss of coordination**

- General inflammation
- High blood pressure
- High triglyceride levels (fats in the blood)
- Sticky platelets (causes clotting)
- Increased risk of cancer.

Some years ago I went to a seminar by Udo Erasmus, who is arguably the world's leading expert on fats. I was more than impressed by his delivery, and the way he explained the nature and importance of essential fatty acids in the diet was truly inspirational. If you think you may have an EFA deficiency, or would like more information on the scientific nature of EFAs and other nutrients then I would recommend his book, *Fats That Heal, Fats That Kill.* If I could only ever own one nutrition book, this would be it. It is the absolute 'fat bible'!

If you suffer from any of the more serious conditions listed above, or in particular, if you have ever suffered from cancer, then the information you need to regain health is beyond the scope of this book, but Udo's book, and his range of oils, are absolutely essential for you. Visit www.udoschoice.co.uk for more information, and to see a range of his outstanding products.

By using the colour code system in chapter 12, you will learn how to choose the right foods to ensure that you get a good intake of EFAs, and enjoy all the health benefits that entails. If you have been deficient for some time, it can take several weeks, or in extreme cases even months, to see visible changes on the exterior (skin), because the cells inside will always heal first. Once again,

I remind you of the man who chose the penny and sat back and enjoyed his compound interest!

Protein

Protein is the element of food that gives it – and us when we eat it – structure. It is contained in meat and animal products, but also in non-animal foods such as seeds, nuts and all pulses. Protein should make up approximately 20–25 per cent of your total dietary/daily intake. It is a vital component of all living cells. After water, protein is the most abundant nutrient in our bodies, but despite its importance, the reason you need less protein than carbohydrate or fat is because, unlike the other fats and carbs, protein is not used for energy production. Therefore it doesn't need to be replaced as often because it stays in the body for much longer. Protein has a calorific value of 4 calories per gram.

Protein is made up of amino acids, which are like building blocks. If we put them together in the right way, we can make whatever we need for our bodies out of these blocks. Think of it this way: we have 26 letters in our alphabet, which we use in different combinations to make up all the words we need. But to make a word, we need to include a vowel to give it structure. In the same way, we use a variety of amino acids to build healthy cells and structures, but we must include one of the eight *essential amino acids* in order to make a complete structure.

There are a few fundamental differences in the way the body handles protein compared to fat or carbohydrates.

Protein takes a long time to digest and therefore keeps us satisfied for a long time, whereas carbohydrate digestion begins in the mouth. Protein can only be digested in the stomach because it's much harder to break down. The stomach is a sealed sac which contains a special acid called hydrochloric acid that is required to break down protein. The stomach lining is covered in a coating of thick, phlegm-like fluid that protects it against the harmful effects of the acid. If the acid does escape to other areas outside the stomach, it causes burns and ulcers, so there are valves at the entrance and exit of the stomach to prevent this from happening. Both fat and carbohydrates need to pass through the stomach to be digested in the intestines, as they need different alkaline enzymes to break them down.

How Much Protein Is Enough?

There has been a lot of controversy in recent years about the benefits or otherwise of the 'high-protein, low-carb' diet – and the many other diets that are variations on the same theme. As you know, certain aspects of this regime are helpful, but if taken to extremes, they can be terribly harmful. Protein contains nitrogen, which the body converts into ammonia and then urea; this is excreted by the kidneys. This highly acidic process can be undertaken safely all the time the correct amount of protein is being eaten, but if the diet is consistently high in protein the kidneys can begin to suffer from the effects of the extra work they need to do. This can be felt as anything from a slight backache to – at worse – full kidney failure.

A long-term high-protein diet has other negative effects. For example, the body becomes too acidic and to combat this, it extracts calcium (which is very alkaline) from the bones and dumps it into the bloodstream to compensate. Over time, this can lead to osteoporosis, as well as an increased risk of heart disease, because circulating calcium makes the blood very viscous (scratchy) and can damage artery walls. High-protein diets also prohibit the intake of fruits and vegetables (which is *not* a good thing); although they do also limit high-GI refined carbs (which *is* a good thing).

In the previous chapter we looked at why you need to increase the amount of muscle tissue (LBM) in your body in order to maximize the amount of fat you can burn. However, this is *not* done by eating vast amounts of protein. Your body decides how much protein to use for muscle growth (as opposed to many other things) based purely on how often and how much you use your muscles. If you sat on your bed and consumed vast numbers of protein shakes, you would still get fat.

Your body is smart – it has an intelligence beyond comprehension. It operates solely on feedback, so if your muscles are not sending messages to your brain saying, 'I need to be stronger', then no extra protein will be delivered for muscle growth. If, however, you are exercising and challenging your muscles *and* eating good quality protein, then your muscles, and therefore your metabolic rate, will increase.

In terms of diet, the problem is that many foods that contain protein also contain fat. Which is why, as you will see, they are grouped together on the colour code system. In fact, there are very few foods that contain protein that don't also contain fat (typically oils and butter). Relying solely on meat to get your protein is not a healthy way to eat a balanced diet. Whether you are a vegetarian or a meat eater, you must ensure that you consume vegetables and grains and non-meat sources of good quality protein such as the following:

- Quinoa (a grain/fruit from South America)
- Soya (e.g. tofu)
- Beans
- Lentils
- Fresh, uncooked seeds
- Fresh, uncooked nuts
- Wholegrains
- Low-fat dairy products (preferably organic).

Carbohydrate

A carbohydrate is something that contains glucose. This may mean it's almost entirely glucose, or that it contains glucose and other nutrients. The easiest way to define a carbohydrate is that 'it doesn't have a face'. In other words, it's grown in or on the soil and doesn't come from animals. Years ago, carbohydrates were defined as 'simple' or 'complex' – this simply referred to the size of the molecules. We have now developed a much better understanding of the molecular make-up of carbohydrates and how they behave in our bodies.

Carbohydrates as a food group contain many different substances, including:

- Glucose
- Fructose (fruit sugar)
- Vitamins
- Minerals
- Fibre
- Phytochemicals
- Enzymes
- Prebiotics.

When we talk about carbohydrates we usually think first of glucose and 'sugar'. We've already explored the importance of maintaining healthy blood sugar levels, and understanding how we digest and absorb carbohydrates. In this section we are going to look specifically at the foods that enable you to do that.

Sugar

There are two kinds of sugar – glucose, which is an immediately usable form of energy – and fructose (fruit sugar) – which has to be taken to the liver and converted to glucose before it can be used for energy. This is a crucial difference, because glucose raises blood sugar instantly and fructose has a more moderate effect. Glucose has a calorific value of 4 calories per gram; the same as protein, and less than half the calories of fat, which has 9 calories per gram. Providing you eat low GI foods (see below), you can eat more food in terms of weight and actually eat fewer calories. However, because it's so easy to overeat refined, fat-free or fat-reduced foods, you can easily eat twice as much as you would do if the food contained fat. This is why so many people struggle to lose weight on the low-fat diet.

For several years, I was consultant to Rosemary Conley and worked hand-in-hand with her to create and build the RC Diet and Fitness Clubs. One of my jobs was to support the franchisees (whom I trained) and help them if one of their members wasn't losing weight. I can't tell you how many food diaries I saw that were virtually fat free, but the member was eating so much fat-free food that they overcompensated for the fat calories they had removed with starchy carbohydrates. They would have a huge plate of pasta with only a tiny amount of Bolognese sauce because they saw the pasta as fat-free therefore not fattening. They ate so much fat-free pasta, rice, and bread (without butter!) that it caused a glucose spike and their bodies released extra insulin to convert the excess to fat. They got fat without even eating fat! Even healthy food will lead to weight gain if you constantly eat more than you need! It's all about balance.

The Glycemic Index (GI)

GI is an invaluable tool. It's simply an index, or a list, that assigns to a food a numerical value that represents how quickly it is absorbed into the bloodstream. They key to understanding GI is to be aware that it determines the rate of digestion – it's that simple. Foods that speed quickly through your digestive system (such as refined foods) don't suppress appetite, whereas foods that reach the small intestine before they are fully digested (such as fibre-rich foods) stimulate the secretion of messenger signals to the brain saying, 'full up!' and you naturally stop eating because the hunger signal is switched off.

What you eat (not just how much) affects your appetite; if you stay fuller longer, then you are less susceptible to cravings and generally eat less. If you choose foods that are medium or low GI then you are assured of eating foods that take longer to digest and help suppress hunger. In addition, nature has given us another benefit associated with these foods: they are often rich in nutrients and contain many other vital components, including vitamins, minerals and fibre. When it comes to 'filling power', all foods are not equal, and that's what the GI helps us to understand.

Dr Jennie Brand-Miller is an Australian nutritionist known as 'The Queen of the Glycemic Index', and her excellent book, *The Low GI Diet,* led to a deluge of copycat diets and books. In a similar way to what happened with the high-protein diet, many of these took a sound concept and took it to extremes. I have had clients come to me saying they are 'not allowed' to eat fruit. This is absolute rubbish. If you want to learn more about the GI diet from the real expert, then Dr Brand-Miller should be your only source.

All About Antioxidants

The colour code system in the next chapter takes full account of the principles of the GI. You will see that there are two classifications for carbohydrates: **PINK** being the higher GI foods that should be eaten in moderation (or some not at all!) and **GREEN**, which represents fruit and vegetables – these can be eaten freely. Many people mistakenly stop eating fruit, thinking it causes a rush in blood sugar, but this is not the case as its sugar – fructose – goes to the liver first to be converted into glucose. There are very few exceptions to this rule – such as dates, some grapes, and melons – but if you eat these as part of a fruit salad with more fibrous fruit, they don't pose a problem. You would need to eat a very large portion of grapes to cause an insulin spike.

Fruits and vegetables are also an essential source of antioxidants; these are precious substances that protect against cancer and also slow down the ageing process. You don't have to be an expert to learn which foods contain antioxidants; there is a very simple guideline:

If it's fresh and colourful, it contains antioxidants.

The good news is that foods containing antioxidants are also typically low GI. For example, sweet potatoes are much lower on the GI than white potatoes, and are also rich in antioxidants.

Other foods high in antioxidants include the following:
- **Carrots**
- **Broccoli**
- **Cabbage**

- All berries: strawberries, cranberries, etc.
- Peppers (all colours)
- Watercress
- Cauliflower
- Melon
- Spinach
- Peas
- Tomatoes
- Lemons.

You'll notice that many of these foods are on the 'banned' list on the high-protein diet. This is further evidence of how dangerous this approach can be.

Mabel's Journal

After the really interesting chapters on hormones and fat cells I was well up for reading this bit, and finally getting to the 'diet' (I know it's not a diet!!). Yet again, I was reminded of how I have used food as a reward for so much of my life. It strikes me that the food itself rewards ME, but only if I eat the right stuff. When I do, my reward is that I'm going to be slimmer and much healthier. That's the only way food is going to be a reward for me from now on.

Note to self: I will never use food as a reward, but I will let the right foods reward me.

When I read the last few chapters, I was a bit surprised to learn the balance of foods that we need. I didn't know we needed so much fat – I've always thought of fat as a bad thing. Looked at my dinner tonight to see if I'm getting the balance right. Had a pork chop (protein and fat) with mashed sweet potatoes (carbs – higher GI) and vegetables (still carbs, but lower GI). So I think I'm getting there, I keep reminding myself that I need good quality protein and carbs that do not cause a sugar spike; I think it's starting to make sense!

I've heard of the glycemic index – I thought it meant no grapes or melon!! Some of the girls in the office did a diet where they weren't allowed fruit. Madness!!

Made a list to help me when I go food shopping: I'm going to type it up and print it out for safekeeping! Might even put a copy in the cupboard in the kitchen :o)

Eat More	Eat Less
Fresh seeds – take to work	Red meat (cut off fat if I do eat it)
Fresh nuts (mix with seeds)	Hard cheese (get soft organic if possible)
Fish (e.g. tuna steak)	Fizzy drinks (try lemon barley water)
Vegetables – some raw	
Salad – use vegetables in salad	
Organic milk/dairy	

Chapter 12

THE COLOUR CODE SYSTEM

My goal in this section is to give you enough nutritional information for you to be able to create a 'diet' that works for you. The simple colour code system that follows is designed to focus on getting you healthy and balancing your hormones so you become a natural fat burner. With this system *you* get to choose the foods you eat and you can create your own diet based on what you know will work. As you know by now, no two people are exactly the same, so, based on how you feel, and how much weight you want to lose, you can adapt it slightly to find the right combination for you.

The colour code system is slightly different for the first two weeks, in the form of the Healthy Starter Plan (see p.207). This is designed to give you a great start by boosting liver function and stabilizing blood sugar more quickly; as you know from the previous chapters these are vital components of weight loss, and following this system will maximize your fat-burning potential in the medium and longer term. If you find that your progress slows at any time you can simply return to the Healthy Starter Plan to give yourself a boost, as it's only slightly different from the regular colour code system in this chapter.

If you find that the Healthy Starter Plan works well for you and your energy levels are good, you can stay on it for longer than two weeks, or maybe use it for most days and the regular system for others. *You* are taking control of what you eat and what works for you. It's empowering, isn't it!

I have only two 'golden rules' when it comes to food:

1. **Never use any food as a reward or a treat.** Eat for one reason only: because your body needs fuel. And give it the best quality fuel possible. If you enjoy consuming the fuel, then so much the better! Eating is a great social activity and should be enjoyed, but eating out doesn't have to mean getting fat – you can apply my guidelines wherever you are.

2. **Never ban yourself from eating something.** This will only make you want it more. That doesn't mean I'm not going to say, 'don't have' certain foods – in a few cases I'm going to say just that! But I'm talking in general terms, and of course what I'm really saying is, 'If you have these foods other than once in a blue moon, you will get or stay fat.' You make the final choice as to what you put in your mouth, not me.

The colour code system is made up of four food groups:

GREEN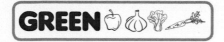

Vegetables and fruit and most foods that grow in the soil. Range from medium–low GI, with a high nutritional content (including antioxidants); they also contain good levels of fibre.

PINK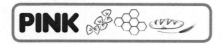

Starchy carbohydrates – i.e. all grains and related products (pasta, bread, rice, cereals, etc.) plus potatoes. Range from high–moderate GI foods with a moderate–good nutritional value, to high GI foods with a low nutritional value.

BLUE

Fats and proteins, including fish, meat, dairy, nuts, seeds, oils. Range from high nutritional value foods containing good levels of EFAs to low nutritional value saturated fatty acids.

RED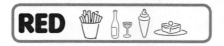

Sweets, cream, ice-cream, alcohol, sugar, refined honey, pastries (sweet or savoury), cakes, crisps, deep-fried chips, high-fat takeaway meals, etc. Food that has no nutritional benefit whatsoever – just empty calories.

In some of the groups, you will see a * beside a food. This indicates that it also contains strong elements of another group. For example, lentils are classified as (GREEN) because they grow as beans in the soil and are a good source of fibre. When they are harvested and the lentils are separated from the plant, they are low on the glycemic index. But they are also an excellent source of protein (BLUE), so they cross two food groups. Another example is dried fruit, which is also (GREEN), but has a higher GI than fresh fruit as much of the flesh and fluid has been removed, leaving mainly glucose; this has a * (PINK) next to it.

You can use the arrows to gauge which foods are the best choice; wherever possible, reduce or avoid the choices at the bottom of the arrows and choose instead from the foods higher up the list.

How Much Should You Eat?

Each section has an individual guideline for portion sizes. *How much* you eat is as important as *what* you eat. Remember I told you about all the low-fat dieters who got fat? Many of them ate more calories than they needed just because they weren't fat calories. You must become more aware of just how much you eat – even 'healthy' calories will make you fat if you eat too many of them.

You must use your own common sense and intelligence here. After all, you'll be kidding yourself if you think you can carry on eating as much as you are now and lose weight. It's also important to note that the speed at which you eat influences how *much* you eat.

Studies have shown that people who chew their food more, and who put their cutlery down in between each mouthful, eat less overall (estimates show this can be up to 200 calories less per meal!).

Be aware that a portion size isn't designed to make you 'full up' – it's designed to satisfy and nourish you. There's a big difference between being satisfied, i.e. eating enough, and being full up. When you are full up, the uncomfortable sensation you get is your stomach telling you it is over-distended (stretched). Unfortunately, people get used to this sensation and programme themselves, or anchor it, to be the feeling they think they should get after every meal, and they don't stop eating until they get it. Next time you feel uncomfortable after eating, think about how much you've had and make a mental note to listen to your body.

You can do this by understanding how the 'feedback' system between your stomach and your brain works. Your stomach has sensors all around it that send messages to the brain depending on how much it is distending. When you are tuned in to this sensation, your brain uses this signal to turn off hunger. Unfortunately, the sensation can be quite subtle and it's easy to ignore, especially if you eat quickly. By the time you process the signal you've already eaten overeaten and it's too late. Imagine your stomach as an empty balloon, but with a thick elastic band around it. As you blow the balloon up, the elastic band becomes tighter and you can see the amount of air that you can comfortably put into the balloon before the elastic band snaps. If your stomach snapped like the elastic band when you over-filled it, you'd be in trouble! Unlike the balloon though, your stomach can be severely overstretched before you physically have to stop eating.

Tip
· · · ·

Try this visual reminder to stop yourself from overeating. Wear a brightly coloured elastic band every time you eat to remind yourself that your stomach can carry on stretching long after you have had enough to eat. I've often given new clients a band and asked them not to take it off for two weeks (except to sleep). It's a simple technique but it has worked for many people – why not try it and see if it works for you.

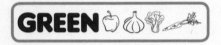

GREEN

Cruciferous (leafy) green vegetables

All raw vegetables (including peppers)

Lightly cooked (or steamed) vegetables

Avocados * **BLUE** also a good source of EFAs

Lentils * **BLUE** also a good source of protein

Beans * **BLUE** also a good source of protein

Tofu * **BLUE** also a good source of protein

Frozen peas

Corn

All crunchy, not over-ripe fruit (e.g. apples and pears)

Soft fruits (including bananas) and berries

Fruit juice (unsweetened)

Dried fruit * **PINK** high GI

Portion Sizes

All portion sizes given are guidelines, as individual body mass determines how many calories you need.

- Raw vegetables – unlimited
- Cooked vegetables – up to a large mug full
- Fruit: hand-held, e.g. bananas, apples, pears, oranges, etc. – one piece; for avocado, half
- Berries – 2–3 heaped tablespoons
- Lentils/beans – 1 cup full (uncooked)
- Fruit juice – approximately 250 ml (9 fl oz): best diluted with water
- Dried fruit – small, level palm full (best eaten with something from **BLUE** group, such as nuts)

General guidelines

1. For the first two weeks, while you are on the Healthy Starter Plan (see p.207), aim to have at least one raw vegetable-based meal (can be served with lightly cooked lean meat or fish) per day. Have unlimited amounts of raw or lightly cooked vegetables, but aim for a *minimum* of three portions per day.
2. After the Healthy Starter plan, make sure you continue to eat moderate amounts of crunchy fruit (2–3 portions per day).
3. Eat 1–2 portions of soft fruit per day.
4. Dilute concentrated (unsweetened) fruit juice with water.

5. Eat as many different, brightly coloured vegetables and fruits as possible, e.g. green/orange/yellow/red – this will ensure a good balance of vitamins and minerals, as well as maximizing your intake of antioxidants.

6. Use raw spinach and watercress in salads rather than just lettuce leaves.

7. Reduce the amount of meat you use in dishes such as curries and casseroles and replace with vegetables, beans or lentils. For example, make a chicken and vegetable curry in place of a chicken curry.

8. Total portions from the **GREEN** section per day: 7–10.

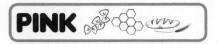

PINK

Quinoa

Barley

Oats

Brown rice/wild rice (al dente)

Basmati rice (al dente)

Sweet potato

Muesli (no added sugar)

Couscous

Unrefined cereals (no added sugar)

Multigrain breads (with 'bits')

Rye bread

Fruit loaf

Wholemeal pasta (al dente)

White pasta (al dente)

Rye crispbreads

Chapatis

Gluten-free bread

Rice cakes

Wholemeal pitta bread

Corn wraps

Tortilla wraps

Brown bread

White pitta bread

Polenta

Bagels

Muffins

White bread

White potato

Unrefined honey

Waffles

Pizza

Sugar   * (RED) (empty calories)

Portion Sizes

All portion sizes given are guidelines, as individual body mass determines how many calories you need.

- Quinoa, oats, rice, pasta, polenta, couscous, etc. – 1 cup full (uncooked)

- Sweet potato – 1 medium/large
- White potato – 1 medium/large or 4–5 small new potatoes
- Bread (including fruit loaf) – 2 medium-cut slices (multigrain) or 1 chapati
- Bagels/pitta breads/waffles/muffins/wraps, etc. – 1
- Honey and sugar – 1 teaspoon
- Cereals – 1 small bowl muesli (weight varies depending on ratio of ingredients: *nuts are heavier than oat flakes)*, plus added fruit (any kind)
- Processed cereals – 250 g (9 oz)
- Pizza – 1 small (7-inch)
- Crispbreads/rice cakes – 2
- Sugar/honey – 1 teaspoon

General Guidelines

1. During the Healthy Starter Plan, have no more than 1–2 portions of (**PINK**) per day.
2. After the plan, 2–3 portions per day is fine *as long as you choose from the top of the arrow, i.e. the lower GI options.*
3. Avoid or reduce the foods listed at the base of the arrow (i.e. from muffins and below).
4. You must *not* exclude (**PINK**) altogether, as without them it's difficult to get the amount of glucose your cells need. The key is to choose the right ones (i.e. the ones at the top of the arrow).
5. Total portions of (**PINK**) foods per day: 1–2.

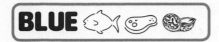

BLUE

Fish (raw or lightly cooked and if possible, wild not farmed)

Udo's Oil (use in salad dressings or as a supplement)

Lean meat (preferably organic)

Fresh, uncooked nuts

Fresh, uncooked seeds

Extra-virgin olive oil

Eggs (organic if possible)

Cow's milk (organic if possible)

Rice milk

Soy milk

Yoghurt (low sugar)

Soft cheese

Hard cheese

Vegetable oils (for cooking)

Butter

Margarine

Portion Sizes

Of all the food groups, the portion sizes vary more with **BLUE** than any other colour. This makes sense when you look at the range of foods included, many of which contain fat and/or protein. So the portion may be as small as some milk in your tea, or as big as a steak for your dinner! So you obviously need to exercise some common sense when choosing from this group. All sizes are guidelines, because individual body mass determines how many calories you need.

- Meat and fish – women 113–170 g (4–6 oz); men 170–226 g (6–8 oz)
- Fresh, uncooked nuts – a palm full
- Fresh, uncooked seeds (crack the husks before eating to release the oils) – 1 dessert spoonful
- Oils – 1–2 teaspoons per serving, e.g. in dressings mixed with vinegar
- Milk (all kinds) – approximately 250 ml (9 fl oz)
- Eggs – 1 large
- Yoghurt – 1 small pot
- Soft cheese 56–113 g (2–4 oz) as part of main meal or up to 55 g (1–2 oz) as a snack
- Hard cheese 56–113 g (2–4 oz) as part of main meal or up to 55 g (1–2 oz) as a snack
- Butter – use sparingly
- Margarine – use sparingly

General guidelines

1. For the Healthy Starter Plan (see p.207) limit the amount of red meat, or exclude it altogether in favour of lightly cooked fish. Have a handful of fresh nuts and seeds *every* day, and use unrefined extra-virgin olive or Udo's Oil for salad dressings.

2. Have a **BLUE** food with *every* meal – it will keep you satisfied for longer.

3. Do *not* eat only (**BLUE**) foods – i.e. a high-protein diet. Always combine your overall intake of blues with (**GREEN**) and/or (**PINK**) foods.

4. Have meat no more than once per day (and have two meat-free days per week).

5. Choose low-fat options wherever possible – including lean meat and skimmed or semi-skimmed milk and dairy produce.

6. Hard cheese has much more saturated fatty acids than soft cheese, so moderate the amount of hard cheese you eat and mix with softer options.

7. Use soft, lower-fat cheeses for making sauces, or choose a very strong hard cheese so you need only a little to get the cheesy taste you require.

8. Watch out for low-fat options in the supermarket – they are often full of sugar to replace the taste of the fat.

9. If you are vegetarian, you need to pay particular attention to the quality of the blues selected and *not* rely solely on cheese and other dairy products for your protein. Revisit the (**GREEN**) section and look at beans, pulses and lentils, which also have a (**BLUE**) star: you should have at least 1–2 portions of these per day.

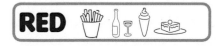
RED

These are all the foods that have little or no nutritional value. It's not possible to list every single unhealthy food here, so once again use your common sense and don't deceive yourself!

- All confectionery
- Potato crisps
- Pastries (sweet or savoury)
- Alcohol
- Canned, sugary drinks
- High-fat takeaway meals
- Cream/ice-cream
- Most cakes and biscuits

General Guidelines

Let's make it really clear: *you are not on a diet!* So that means nothing is 'forbidden' and it's OK to have *anything* on the (RED) list *sometimes*; that is occasionally, *not* every day. Now you have already learnt, and you can re-learn as you re-read the chapters that have helped you the most, that with a combination of changing your mind, and what you eat, cravings can literally disappear. Your desire for unhealthy foods can and will diminish, at your command!

The problem with these (RED) foods is that you don't see the fat immediately you eat them, so one takeaway doesn't mean you can't get into your jeans the next day. This is how we allow ourselves to overeat, because we cannot see the damage quickly enough to fully associate it with the foods we eat. But now you have accepted that what you ate made you fat. I know you have, otherwise you wouldn't have got to this part of the book. So give yourself a huge pat on the back, and one from me!

If you find that you are having some (**RED**) foods every day, then go back and re-read the chapters that you feel are the most relevant to you. As a very general guideline, aim to eat no more than 2–3 (**RED**) foods per week *maximum*. Please remember, though, that (**RED**) foods are not compulsory and this is the only colour group that it's OK not to have any of!

Use the information in both the psychological and nutrition parts of the book to achieve your goal. This really is a *mind and body approach*, and no other system has ever fully offered that, so make the most of all you have learnt and choose to make the changes that will give you the healthy body that is your birthright. Go and claim it now!

The Healthy Starter Plan

For the first two weeks of using the colour code system, I recommend that you follow the Healthy Starter Plan I'm about to give you, as it will take the stress off your liver and other systems. This way, your body can establish a level of health that will enable you to burn more fat more effectively – and you know from the earlier chapters how beneficial this will be. You may or may not lose a significant amount of weight over this two-week period (although many people do experience a significant drop in weight, especially if they are prone to bloating and fluid retention). The goal is to establish for you a healthy physiology that will enable you to lose more weight in the medium and longer term, so it is well worth the effort.

The Healthy Starter Plan is not a strict detox – and it isn't that different from the general recommendations in the last chapter – but it is a more disciplined way of eating and cleansing to give your body a boost and maximize your future progress. Although there are recommendations within the colour code system as to what to eat, the Healthy Starter Plan is more about *what not to eat for two weeks*. Use the Daily Check Lists on p.223 to monitor your progress and stay on track. Either copy the template there or download it from www.powertochange.me.uk by clicking on *Think More, Eat Less* on the home page and using 'Positive Attitude' as the password.

While you are on the plan, it is important to avoid the following:

- Alcohol
- Caffeine
- Tobacco
- Foods from the (RED) group
- Processed and packaged foods
- Wheat (whenever possible).

Support for your Liver

You will find stopping caffeine a lot easier if you cut down gradually over a week; if you are a caffeine craver, stopping it straight off will result in you having headaches and feeling rough for three to five days. This runs counter to everything you can achieve on this programme – I want you to feel good and build positive anchors not negative ones – so stop caffeine at your own pace and gradually replace it with herbal or fruit teas. Here's a list of some liver-cleansing herbs and foods that are available as teas, drinks or supplements from your health shop. They can also all be blended together to make a juice that will support and cleanse the liver:

- **Milk thistle**
- **Dandelion**
- **Artichoke leaves**
- **Pomegranate (not processed)**
- **Beetroot (not pickled)**
- **Grapefruit**
- **Berries**
- **Rosemary**
- **Liquorice.**

General Guidelines

1. Meat – have at *least* two meat-free days a week, and if practical or possible, buy organic. If using red meat, cook it rare or medium rare as this is easier to digest.

2. Fish – eat oily fish (not farmed) at least twice a week.

3. Dairy – choose organic milk and cheese if practical or possible. Avoid hard cheese in favour of soft cheese and have a *maximum* of two portions of dairy per day – for example one portion of milk in cereal and one portion of cheese in a salad or meal.

4. Drink plenty of water in addition to the drinks suggested, so you can flush out toxins.

5. Consume lots of high-fibre foods (you'll automatically be doing this because you'll be eating raw and lightly cooked vegetables) as this will aid the clearing process.

6. Aim to eat a minimum of three portions of raw vegetables per day, either in salads or chopped as snacks.

7. Add as many cruciferous (leafy) vegetables to your meals as possible. Boil them in a little water, or steam them.

8. Eat foods that contain EFAs, such as olives, avocados, uncooked nuts and seeds (broken to release the oils), fish (raw sushi fish without the rice is ideal). Or Udo's Oil (see supplements section on p.233).

9. Eat three times per day – *do not skip meals*, because you need to maintain a constant blood sugar to avoid stressing the liver.

10. Avoid bread (absolutely *no* white bread) and all wheat products whenever possible.

11. Use quinoa instead of rice, potatoes (except sweet potatoes, which are fine) and pasta.

Sample Meals For The Healthy Starter Plan

Breakfast

- Take a large cup or a small mug of frozen (or fresh if in season) berries and blend them with an organic yoghurt in a simple hand blender.

- Homemade juice using beets, cabbage, apples, celery or similar fruit and vegetables.
- Organic, sugar-free muesli with chopped apples.

Lunch

- Homemade vegetable soup.
- Salad (including chopped or grated raw vegetables) with fish or lean meat and homemade salad dressing (e.g. extra-virgin olive oil, or Udo's Oil with balsamic vinegar, mustard powder and a light squeeze of lemon or lime).

Dinner

- Salad (as above).
- Stir-fry of crispy vegetables (lightly cooked in oil) with garlic, ginger, fresh chillies, etc. (add other spices to taste), with lightly cooked fish or meat. Serve with quinoa.
- Lentil and vegetable bake or casserole served with leafy green vegetables.

Snacks

- Raw vegetables and hummus.
- Apples and other crunchy fruit.
- Homemade smoothies.
- Fresh, uncooked nuts and seeds (crack the husks to release the oil).

Drinks

- Fruit teas, green tea, white tea, hot or cold water with lemon slices, any diluted, unsweetened fruit juice.

After the first two weeks are over, you can begin to adapt the system to suit your own likes and dislikes; don't eat something just because it's healthy – whatever nutrient it contains can almost certainly be found in something else. I wanted to 'train' myself to like green and white tea, so every time I tasted them I closed my eyes and thought of a taste I really enjoyed, and anchored it to the taste of the green and white tea. After a few attempts it worked well and I drink these teas every day. However, for some reason my taste buds just will not accept the taste of olives, no matter what I try and anchor it to! So I use unrefined olive oil and make sure I get plenty of EFAs from other sources. Although food is medicine, it shouldn't taste like medicine!!!

Exercise

During the two weeks of the Healthy Starter Plan, aim to be active, but not aggressive, with your exercise regime. If you are a non-exerciser, aim to walk briskly or swim for at least 20–30 minutes at least four times a week (or a little less if this is too much for you). If you are already a regular exerciser then be sure to maintain your usual level, but don't increase it during these two weeks. Remember: the aim of the plan is to get healthy! Part of that process is to allow your body to rest and recover and enable the nutrients you are taking in to work to best effect. Once your body has done that, it will respond much better when you introduce some new and more challenging activities, especially those that increase muscle tone (LBM) such as resistance training – which may be going to a gym or just cycling or walking up hills instead of staying on the flat!

Mabel's Journal

Have finally got to the 'diet' only to find out it is NOT a diet!!! Such a relief! I can totally see how this will be easy to follow. Some nice surprises, too: I love avocado and previous slimming clubs and diets have 'banned' it!! How awful to ban a food that's so healthy! It's the same with grapes too: what have I been doing??! This is so refreshing: everything makes perfect sense.

When I made dinner tonight I tried to imagine my plate divided into three colours to get the balance right. I had chicken (BLUE), new potatoes (PINK) and carrots and peas (GREEN). Took a mental picture of this and need to apply it to everything. I think this is on the right lines! Doesn't feel like a diet at all.

Some things I need to work on, though, so I'm going to make another list!!

1. How to get raw vegetables into my diet – use in snacks, dips, or chopped in salads.
2. How to get more EFAs into my diet – fresh nuts and seeds for snacks. Google some nice tuna recipes!!
3. How to get plenty of fibre – raw veg (above), crunchy fruit, e.g. apples (also good for liver), berries (could blend with yoghurt and Udo's Oil for 'super nutritious' breakfast?). Make some homemade muesli or buy a low-sugar variety.
4. Good quality proteins every meal – fish (not farmed!!), lean meat, beans and lentils (make my own vegetable and lentil soup).

Things to Stop!

1. *No more white bread!*
2. *Maximum of two REDS per week (some weeks I've not even been having that, so that will be easy!)*
3. *Alcohol only when I am out and then in moderation (that will be my most of my REDS!!). Have spritzers and drink slower. Come to think of it, will eat slower as well! I tried the elastic band exercise and only needed to wear it for a few days – it really made me think about not stretching my stomach!*
4. *Already stopped scabs and slimey, pukey chocolate. (GO ME!!!!!)*

Made a list of everything I've eaten today to see if I'm on the right lines. Going to do the Healthy Starter Plan next week as madly busy at work this week and want to plan it properly!

- *Breakfast – muesli (PINK) with yoghurt and spoonful of Udo's Oil (BLUE), chopped apple and half a banana (GREEN).*
- *Lunch – wholemeal wrap (PINK) with watercress, spinach and iceberg lettuce and sliced tomatoes (GREEN) plus feta cheese and brie (BLUE) and balsamic dressing.*
- *Afternoon snack – a large apple with some walnuts.*
- *Dinner – spaghetti Bolognese. Spaghetti (PINK), Bolognese sauce made with lean minced beef (BLUE), plus chopped carrots, courgettes, tomatoes and peppers (GREEN), served with mixed green leaf salad.*
- *Drinks – 4 fruit teas, 1 coffee, 2 bottles of water.*

Been following the colour code system for three days and definitely finding it easier than I thought. The Daily Check Lists are really helping to keep me on track – I am seeing every food as a colour! It's so simple!!

~~~~~~~~~~~~~~~~~~~~~

Had girls' night out on Saturday at a Chinese restaurant. I ordered steamed fish in black bean sauce with steamed veg and just had a spoonful of Julie's fried rice (I didn't want a whole portion). It was yummy! Drank half as much as I normally would have; the spritzer routine is working really well, and I didn't feel at all unsociable. Really getting used to people telling me how well I look, and my 18s are definitely getting too loose. It has only been seven weeks since I started – that's 1½ dress sizes already, and I genuinely don't feel as if I'm dieting. (That's because I'm not – has the penny finally dropped!?)

Energy levels are higher than ever – I can run for 12 minutes now and fast walk for 10 and I actually enjoy going to the gym once a week. Keep visualizing my muscles getting fitter and burning more fat! Still doing the TFT triangle and visualizing with my statements every day. It's becoming a way of life!!

~~~~~~~~~~~~~~~~~~~~~

I decided after reading the nutrition section to go back and re-read the chapter on hormones again, which makes even more sense now. I really do want to give myself a big boost. Now that the party weekend is over, it will be easier to focus on the Healthy Starter Plan. Doesn't look that different from the colour code system, just fewer pinks and no reds; I've pretty much stopped all the processed stuff anyway so that won't be too difficult. Just need to cut out the coffee. I've already gone from four cups a day to one or two without even being conscious that I'm doing it. Is there some kind of hypnotic suggestion in this book that I'm not aware of, or am I finally being kind to my body!! (About time, it cries!!)

Going to make some time tomorrow to have a play with some new recipes. Need to write shopping list first:

- Green leafy vegetables (whatever is in season and looks good)
- Spinach for spinach soup and salads
- Green salad leaves
- Peppers (all colours)
- Onions (red)
- Lentils
- Sweet potatoes
- Frozen berries
- Organic yoghurt/milk
- Fresh walnuts
- Fresh seeds (health shop?)
- Fresh herbs (dried if can't get fresh – update spice cupboard!)
- Fresh garlic and ginger (chillies?)
- Quinoa
- New hand blender!!!!

~~~~~~~~~~~~~~~~~~~~

The first thing I made was a vegetable soup – it was absolutely delicious! The money I spent on a new blender was well worth it! Never realized how easy it is to make soup. Definitely going to make some more!! Made enough to freeze some for when I don't have as much time. I've even ordered a soup recipe book!!

Had stir-fry veg for dinner; made absolute mountains of it! Just blended chilli, garlic and ginger together with a splash of the ginger drink I got from the health shop to make it a bit more liquid – yum yum!! Cooked some quinoa to go with it; it was OK, though I still prefer rice. Need to Google some quinoa recipes if it's such a healthy food, though!

~~~~~~~~~~

Well, I've been on the Healthy Starter Plan for nearly a week and I'm really starting to notice a change. The first thing is my bloating has all but gone. I am wearing size 16 clothes now and it has only been eight weeks since I started reading the book; I can't quite believe it! Haven't weighed myself yet (as instructed not to!) but don't need to as I'm feeling much better! I'm finding it hard-ish to really keep to 1 PINK a day – it's so easy for those little buggers to creep up on you! But it's only for two weeks so it will be fine. I'm sure I can settle on two per day quite happily after that.

I've been continuing with my exercise – it is so much easier now it's warmer, but I'm not pushing myself too hard. I'm actually doing as I'm told for a change!

~~~~~~~~~~

I'm at the end of the Healthy Starter Plan now, and I actually feel like I could keep going for a bit longer!

Definitely going to stay off bread as much as possible – I didn't realize how many stomach cramps I used to get – until they stopped! Am sure it's the wheat in the bread, so definitely going to limit that. Don't actually fancy a coffee either, so I'm not going to have one just for the sake of it. If I want one later, I'll have it, but will aim to have just one per day, and not every day. I'm being disciplined, but I don't actually _feel_ like I'm being disciplined. It just feels like I'm doing what's right for my body!

Been REALLY focusing on my visualization over the last two weeks – actually imagining going inside my body and watching all these new vitamins repairing my insides and getting everything balanced! Reminds me of a movie I saw years ago where they shrunk a man down, put him in a submarine and inserted him into someone's vein. He travelled around the body! Been a bit like that. I've been seeing fat cells shrinking before my eyes and hormones working together as a team instead of one bullying the other out of action! Sounds nuts but I don't care – it works for me :o)

OMG! I tried a Zumba class today at the gym! Was very nervous going in – worrying about my wobbly bits – but there were all shapes and sizes there, and I felt _really_ good when I noticed some of the 'skinnies' weren't as coordinated as me. And I lasted the full 45 mins. Go me!!

Chapter 13

EVERYDAY EATING

Now that you've given your body a rest and recovery period – possibly from years of abuse or misuse – you can begin to be a little more flexible with your food.

In an ideal world, we would all have a wonderful and plentiful supply of organically farmed, fresh vegetables, and plenty of time off work to relax and de-stress, but for so many of us (I include myself!) that is not the case. So, we have to do the best we can with what we have. Nutritionally, you have a lot of great food available and by buying as much fresh produce as possible, limiting the amount of refined foods you eat, and using the colour code system as your guide, you can look forward to a healthy, slim body and loads more energy.

Putting It All Together

Remember this key fact – you are not on a diet! But you do have to eat for the rest of your life, right? That means you need a system – a way of choosing the right foods that will last you a lifetime. Welcome to the colour code

219

system. I must emphasize again that *you* must take responsibility for what you eat: it's just not possible to design one 'diet' that works for absolutely everyone. But you can use the colour code template to create a lifetime eating plan that will bring you health and energy.

As a basic overview, if you aim for 2 **GREEN**, 1 **BLUE** and a maximum 1 **PINK** (or no pinks) in each meal, then you will be right on track. For snacks, stick to **GREEN** and **BLUE**.

Fat and protein have no GI value and are therefore digested more slowly. This means if you combine something from these food groups (for example some brazil nuts – **BLUE** on the colour code system) with a higher GI food such as a banana **GREEN**, then the overall effect on your digestive system is influenced by the *combined* content of both foods.

Here are some other examples of how this works:

MODERATE GI **PINK**	EAT WITH	PROTEIN/FAT **BLUE**
Jacket potato (preferably sweet potato)	+	Tuna or cheese filling
Pasta (wholewheat)	+	Meat and/or vegetable sauce
Multigrain bread	+	Hummus
Oats (cereal)	+	Yoghurt
Rice (basmati)	+	Mixed bean curry/ casserole
Couscous	+	Meat or bean-based sauce

There are moderate GI alternatives that should always be chosen in preference to the higher GI foods:

HIGH GI	MODERATE GI ALTERNATIVE
White potatoes	Sweet potatoes/yam/sweet corn/beans/ barley/lentils/chickpeas/soya beans (including tofu)
White rice	Quinoa, basmati or brown rice/vermicelli rice noodles/cellophane noodles (the clear ones)
Cereals (refined or processed)	Porridge oats/muesli (sugar-free)
White pasta	Wholewheat pasta (cooked al dente)
Canned spaghetti	Reduced sugar tinned baked beans
White bread	Multigrain and seeded bread/fruit loaf/ chapatis (made with chickpea flour, not wheat), wholemeal wraps

So it can be really simple. For a main meal, just choose a good quality protein such as lean meat, fish or beans (**BLUE**), eat with plenty of lightly cooked vegetables (**GREEN**) and restrict the starchy GI foods to the lowest possible available – have no more than one (**PINK**) serving at any one time.

For snacks, do not have high GI or refined foods – stick to fruit and nuts, or raw vegetable nibbles (crudités) with some low-fat dips such as hummus.

The Daily Check List

I have mentioned several times how beneficial it can be to keep a record of what you eat. In my own studies I found this to be the case, but I also found that having to write everything down is a real nuisance and inconvenience. Everything I have taught you has been to avoid a regime that feels like a diet, so I created the Daily Check List to help you easily monitor what you are eating without having to weigh, measure and write it all down.

Opposite is an example of a Daily Check List or you can download one from my website, www.powertochange. me.uk. Click on the *Think More, Eat Less* link and use the password 'Positive Attitude'.

As you can see, each food group is followed by a series of boxes. Simply tick a box each time you have a food from that particular colour. By the end of the day you will be able to assess at a glance how many of each group you have eaten. It's up to you how long you use these cards for. In chapter 2 you learnt about the process of change – starting with Conscious Competence, just like when you first learnt to drive and had to think about every manoeuvre, and after a while progressing to Unconscious Competence, i.e. driving along safely without even thinking about what you are doing.

If you are changing what you eat massively, you may need to use the Daily Check Lists for at least a month, or until your choices become second nature and you know you are on track without having to monitor it. If you have fewer changes to make, then you may only need to use them for a week or so. As with all of this programme, you

DAILY CHECK LIST

Daily Check List

Date:___/___/___

GREEN (up to 10) FRUIT/VEG

PINK (up to 3) BREAD/PASTA/RICE/CEREAL/POTATO

BLUE (up to 5) MEAT/DAIRY/OILS/NUTS/SEEDS

RED MAX 250 CALS

Exercise today?

YES ☐ NO ☐

Daily Check List

Date:___/___/___

GREEN (up to 10) FRUIT/VEG

PINK (up to 3) BREAD/PASTA/RICE/CEREAL/POTATO

BLUE (up to 5) MEAT/DAIRY/OILS/NUTS/SEEDS

RED MAX 250 CALS

Exercise today?

YES ☐ NO ☐

Daily Check List

Date:___/___/___

GREEN (up to 10) FRUIT/VEG

PINK (up to 3) BREAD/PASTA/RICE/CEREAL/POTATO

BLUE (up to 5) MEAT/DAIRY/OILS/NUTS/SEEDS

RED MAX 250 CALS

Exercise today?

YES ☐ NO ☐

must choose what works for you. Using these cards will accelerate your learning to the Unconscious Competence stage more quickly. Even when you are on track, you can use them again, any time you feel you need a refresher. Even now, I still fill in a Daily Check List to show at my seminars, and it never fails to get me focused.

Everyday Eating Meal Suggestions

Breakfast

- Blend berries (fresh or frozen) with yoghurt and a spoonful of Udo's Oil
- Muesli with yoghurt or milk and chopped fresh fruit
- Porridge with fruit and a spoonful of seeds
- SynerProTein drink (see supplements section p.233)
- Fresh fruit salad with yoghurt, nuts and seeds and a spoonful of Udo's Oil
- Baked beans on multigrain toast with a poached egg
- Bacon, poached eggs and baked beans

Lunch

- Sandwiches or wraps filled with the following:
  - Lean meat with dark green salad leaves (i.e. spinach, rocket, watercress), tomatoes and cucumber
  - Brie with beetroot
  - Tuna or salmon with dark green salad leaves and tomatoes
  - Hummus with dark green salad leaves and tomatoes

- Vegetable soups (see recipes p.227)
- Baked beans or poached eggs on toast
- Organic peanut butter on toast with sliced apple
- Jacket potato with following fillings:
    - Baked beans
    - Cheese
    - Bolognese-type sauce
    - Tuna with salad cream (not mayonnaise)
- Wholewheat crispbreads with following toppings and salad:
    - Cheese
    - Tuna or salmon
- Salad with the following:
    - Dark green salad leaves; chopped, raw peppers; carrots; courgettes; broccoli; corn; beetroot and any other uncooked vegetables; plus sprouts or sprouting beans. Sprinkle with lightly cracked seeds and/or fresh nuts, e.g. walnuts
    - Hummus/cheese/lean meat
    - Dressing: Udo's Oil or extra-virgin olive oil whisked with balsamic or white wine vinegar, mustard powder, a sprinkle of 'season all' spice (or other herbs or spices), and a dash of lemon or lime juice. Adjust the ingredients to get a taste you like.

Dinner
. . . .

- Chilli made with minced meat (or Quorn mince) plus vegetables and beans. Serve with brown basmati rice and a dark green mixed salad.

- Curry made with meat and vegetables, or vegetables and lentils or beans. Serve with basmati rice or a chapati, plus plain yoghurt with mint.

- Shepherd's pie made with minced meat (or Quorn mince) and chopped vegetables topped with sweet potato mash. Serve with extra vegetables.

- Fish pie made with a selection of fish and cooked in white wine and leek sauce with a spoonful of light soft cheese. Top with sweet potato mash and serve with extra vegetables.

- Stir-fry of mixed vegetables with chicken or beef. Serve with quinoa, or rice and salad.

- Salad – see lunch suggestions.

This is not a diet, so I encourage you to adapt the dishes and meals you currently cook using the colour code system as a guide. However, I have asked a good friend of mine, the chef Gerry Sweeney, to give you a few recipes and tips that fit in perfectly with the colour code system if you would like to try something new.

Chicken and Crème Fraîche with Apples and Mushrooms

Serves 4
2 onions, finely chopped
4 chicken breasts
400 ml (14 fl oz) dry cider
100 g (3.5 oz) apple purée
400 g (14 oz) mushrooms, sliced
400 ml (14 fl oz) crème fraîche
30 ml (2 tbsp) olive oil
60 g (2 oz) butter

1. Heat the olive oil and half the butter in a saucepan. Add the onions and chicken breasts and brown all over.
2. Add the cider to the pan and simmer for a few minutes.
3. In a separate pan, fry the mushrooms with the rest of the butter until brown. Drain and then add to the chicken and onions and season. Cook on a low heat for 30 minutes.
4. Add the crème fraîche and apple purée to the pan and cook for a further 10 minutes.
5. Serve in a warmed bowl with pasta or new potatoes.

Country Vegetable Soup

Serves 4
50 g (1.5 oz) dried haricot beans
100 g (3.5 oz) leeks, finely shredded
100 g (3.5 oz) carrots, diced
100 g (3.5 oz) turnip or swede, diced
50 g (1.5 oz) fine beans
100 g (3.5 oz) courgettes
100 g (3.5 oz) broad beans
4 tomatoes, deseeded and chopped
50 g (1.5 oz) tomato purée
50 g (1.5 oz) macaroni
1.5 litres (2.5 pints) vegetable stock
30 ml (2 tbsp) olive oil

1. Soak the haricot beans overnight in cold water.
2. Place the beans in a pot of cold water, bring to the boil and gently simmer for 20 minutes. Remove from the heat and run under cold running water.
3. In a separate pan, heat the olive oil. Add the leeks and sweat for 3 minutes.
4. Add the carrots and turnip or swede and cook for a further 2 minutes.
5. Add the haricot beans, cover with the vegetable stock. Add all other ingredients and cook until tender.
6. Season and serve.

Chef's tip: Liquidize 50 g (1.5 oz) of basil, one garlic clove and 15 ml (1 tbsp) of olive oil. Swirl on top of your soup as a garnish.

Tofu Pâté with Green Peppercorn and Paprika Sauce

Serves 4
For the pâté
100 g (3.5 oz) sunflower seeds
300 g (10 oz) tofu
1 carrot, finely grated
25 g (1 oz) chives, finely chopped
30 ml (2 tbsp) sunflower oil
100 ml (3 fl oz) crème fraîche

1. Liquidize the tofu, sunflower seeds and crème fraîche, and season.
2. Put mixture in a bowl and add the carrot and chives.
3. Place in the fridge until chilled.

For the sauce
400 g (14 oz) can of plum tomatoes
25 g (1 oz) crushed green peppercorns
12 g (half a tbsp) paprika
200 ml (6 fl oz) crème fraîche
Juice of half a lemon

1. Purée the tomatoes, peppercorns and paprika with a hand blender.
2. Place in a pan and heat gently for 5 minutes.
3. Add the crème fraîche and bring to the boil.
4. Add the lemon juice and then pass the sauce through a strainer.
5. Serve cool or chilled with the pâté.

Chef's tip: Serve with sweet potato wedges as a main course, or with crudités as a starter – try peppers, carrot batons or celery sticks.

Salmon Stir-Fry with Thai Spices

Serves 4
4 x 160 g (6 oz) salmon fillets
60 g (2 oz) bean shoots
15 g (half a tbsp) ginger, grated
30 g (1 oz) carrots, finely sliced
30 g (1 oz) celery, finely sliced
30 g (1 oz) courgettes, finely sliced
50 g (1.5 oz) coriander, chopped
Lemon grass – half a stalk
1 red chilli, deseeded and finely chopped
15 ml (1 tbsp) soy sauce
28 g (2 tbsp) toasted sesame seeds
15 ml (1 tbsp) fish stock

1. In a frying pan or wok, fry the salmon with a small amount of olive oil for a couple of minutes each side. Remove from the pan and keep warm.
2. In the same pan or wok, stir-fry the vegetables, bean shoots and ginger for a few minutes. Add the chilli and lemon grass and cook for 5 minutes.
3. Add the fish stock and soy sauce.
4. Add the coriander and put the stir-fry mixture into four warmed bowls.
5. Place the warm salmon fillet on top of the vegetables and sprinkle with the toasted sesame seeds.

Plaice Fillet with Mushrooms and Pak Choi

Serves 4
300 g (10 oz) plaice, cut into goujons
30 ml (2 tbsp) soy sauce
10 g (quarter of a tbsp) cornflour
10 g (quarter of a tbsp) fresh ginger, grated
1 egg white, lightly beaten
1 onion, finely chopped
2 small pak choi – leaves separated
50 g (1.5 oz) mushrooms, sliced
40 ml (1.5 fl oz) fish or chicken stock
2 cloves of garlic, crushed

1. Put the plaice goujons in a small bowl. Add half the soy sauce, ginger and cornflour and stir to combine.
2. Add the egg white, season with salt and pepper and stir again.
3. Remove the goujons from the mixture and shallow fry in olive oil in a frying pan or wok until golden brown. Drain on a piece of kitchen roll.
4. Heat a little more oil in the pan or wok. Add the mushrooms, ginger, onions and garlic and fry for 1 minute.
5. Add the pak choi leaves, stir-fry for 1–2 minutes, or until they have wilted slightly.
6. Blend the remaining cornflour, ginger, soy sauce and stock in a small jug. Pour into the pan/wok and stir-fry for 1–2 minutes.
7. Place the goujons into a serving dish and pour over the mushroom and pak choi sauce.

Chickpea Curry

Serves 4
Splash of olive oil
3 carrots, diced
3 celery stalks, diced
2 onions, roughly chopped
1 leek, roughly chopped
2 fresh chillies, finely chopped
50 g (2 tbsp) curry powder
2 x 400 g (14 oz) cans chopped tomatoes
2 x 400g (14 oz) cans chickpeas
100 g (4 tbsp) tomato purée
2 gloves garlic, minced
A pinch of turmeric
250 ml (8 fl oz) vegetable stock (reduce or add more, depending on desired consistency)

1. Heat the oil in a saucepan. Add all the vegetables, plus the onions, chillies and curry powder. Cook on a low heat for 1 minute
2. Add three-quarters of the vegetable stock, the tomatoes, garlic, tomato purée and turmeric.
3. Bring to the boil and simmer for 10 minutes.
4. With a hand blender, liquidize to a fine sauce, adding the remaining stock (or additional stock) as needed. Cook for a further 10 minutes on a medium heat.
5. Add the chickpeas and cook for a further 5 minutes.
6. Serve in warmed bowls with boiled rice.

Supplements

A question I get asked all the time is, 'Which supplements help weight loss?' You can be forgiven for thinking that a pill or a potion may help because you are constantly being bombarded with advertisements for this or that formula that purports to 'aid weight loss'. The truth is that the best supplements are the ones that promote overall health rather than weight loss – the healthier you are, the easier it is to burn fat.

While making it clear that 'supplement' means *as well as,* not *instead of*, I would recommend the following supplements (which I take myself):

- Super Supplemental Vitamins & Minerals. Visit www.powertochange.me.uk and click on the 'Nature's Sunshine' link on the home page. These can be ordered online and delivered direct to your door.

- Udo's Oil. This can be used as a supplement or drizzled on salads (I stir mine into some yoghurt and then pour it on my cereal), or added to stir-fries after cooking. Available direct to your door from www.udoschoice.co.uk.

- SynerProTein drink – a blend of natural amino acids with the right balance of carbohydrates, this can be used as an occasional meal replacement, or regularly as a breakfast drink. Visit www.powertochange.me.uk, and click on the 'Nature's Sunshine' link on the home page and they can be delivered direct to your door.

- Healthy Starter Pack – a herbal mix to cleanse the liver and other organs and promote bowel health. Visit www.powertochange.me.uk and click on 'Nature's Sunshine'.

Mabel's Journal

I felt REALLY good reading this chapter, as I'm already doing pretty much everything in it! It's a week since I finished the Healthy Starter Plan and I've relaxed it slightly while still holding true to the concept most of the time. I've been out once this week, to an Italian restaurant, and found it much easier to choose good stuff than at the Chinese. Had a gorgeous bit of fish with a lemon butter drizzle and a bowl of veg that did look freshly steamed! Shared a dessert with Deborah, which was some kind of fruit flan; it was nice, and I didn't feel like I needed any more! Only had one spritzer as was driving, so another great night!

Learning how to do this stuff at home is one thing – and I've found that quite easy – but it's been managing to stick to the guidelines when I'm out, or rushed off my feet that's been the most helpful. In the past, when I've been on a diet (I'm NOT on a DIET now!!) and I've gone out, 9 times out of 10 I've fallen completely off the wagon and given up! But now I feel in complete control.

I wrote on my mirror again: 'YOU FREAKIN' ROCK MABEL!' I say that quite a lot, and found myself playing the Black Eyed Peas song on repeat: 'I Gotta Feeling' – that tonight's gonna be a good good night!' It has become my signature tune!! Funny, that was in the first chapter and yet it's still in my mind now. Reminds me when it says, 'I've Gotta Feeling' of how, for the first time in my life, I'm in control of what I think and what I feel. I have free will – and with that comes responsibility. I get that now.

Chapter 14

SETTING YOUR GOAL

Take a moment to think about what you want to achieve on this programme. What is your desired outcome? Is it really just to lose weight, or is to feel different about yourself? Perhaps you want feel in control or more confident? What is it that you think losing weight will bring you? What is your *real* goal?

I often think the word 'goal' is misunderstood in this context. The goal is what you want to achieve, but it is based *entirely* on what you *do*. So, if you make your goal relate to your behaviours, then you will automatically achieve the outcome you want. For example, if you only eat junk food and you want to be size 12, you make your goal not to eat junk food – replacing it with planned cooked meals and snacks. You will then automatically lose weight and reach your desired size 12. When you make the *behaviours* the goal, the weight takes care of itself.

A critical factor in achieving a goal is to be *really clear* about what you want to achieve. To do this you need to write it down, and then create an action plan using tried-and-tested principles in order to achieve it. Have a look back to pp.19–20 at Napoleon Hill's 13 principles. This book has been designed to guide you through these, and if you have completed all the exercises and 'played full-out', then you are well on the way. The final step is to plan your strategy, which you've no doubt been forming as you've read the book.

Creating A Strategy

Step 1: What dress/trouser size do you want to achieve?

I want to be size _____

There is a reason I have put size and not weight, and you will know from the earlier chapters that this is because weight does not take into account body composition. For example, someone like Arnold Schwarzenegger might weigh the same as a sumo wrestler, and both would be classified as 'morbidly obese', but clearly one is fat and the other muscular, so body composition is key.

Step 2: When do you want to achieve it by?

I want to be size _____ by _____

Make sure your desired size and the time frame you have given are realistic. As a guide, you can lose approximately one dress size per month if you go from a starting point of unhealthy eating and inactivity to healthy eating and activity. If your time frame expects a loss of more than one dress size per month, you may need to re-think it, as it's important you know it's genuinely achievable.

On a scale of 1–10, if one is none and 10 is full-out commitment, how much effort are you prepared to put in, starting today? Be honest. You can still get results at 5/10, but of course it will be harder because you are not really embracing the changes wholeheartedly and are more likely to slip back into your old ways. In my own case I would give myself 8.5/10 in terms of the amount of time I devote to healthy eating and activity. I still go out for a slap-up meal sometimes and I don't believe a 'holier than thou' approach works very well for most people. If it's too strict it becomes a diet, and it's unpleasant, so for all the reasons you have learnt in this book, you are likely to self-sabotage. For real success you need to be 8 or above on this programme, and for the first two weeks at least a 10 so you can break some old habits and make a clean start. That's what the Healthy Starter Plan is for.

For the exercise below you will need to refer back to some of the exercises in the earlier chapters. I recommend re-reading some of the psychology chapters now that you have a good understanding of how your body works and what to eat, as you will find your unconscious mind is filling up with ideas about how to combine the behavioural techniques with the colour code system in a way that suits you.

Exercise
· · · · · · · · ·

Get six pieces of A4 paper or card and write the following on them:

1. 1 day
2. 1 week
3. 1 month
4. 3 months
5. 6 months
6. 12 months

Look at the cards and, based on your desired outcome and time frame, make a note of the point at which you will have achieved your new dress size. If it's longer than 12 months, simply add a seventh card.

1. **Now, refer back to the exercises in the earlier chapters of the book and note all the things you want or need to change.** Which of these changes can you commit to doing *within the next 24 hours* in order to make a positive difference in the way you think and behave? Write them on the first piece of paper or card; aim to write at least two things and make sure one is a psychological change (for example, 'Stop telling myself I'm useless and start giving my self positive encouragement') and the other a nutritional change (for example, 'Stop snacking on crisps and get some fresh nuts and seeds or fruit instead').
2. **After you have read the whole of this instruction, place the first piece of paper or card on the floor and stand behind it.** Take a deep breath and step onto it. As you do so, imagine the changes you have written down are being uploaded into your mind. Imagine this is *really* happening, and as you do, create in your mind's eye images of you *doing* these things the next day.

When you have done this fully, step off the paper or card and imagine that day has already happened, and that you already have a day's experience under your belt.

3. **On the second piece of paper or card, write down what you want to change over the next seven days** (in addition to the changes you have already made or implemented on the first day). As before, make sure you include psychological and nutritional changes. In the same way as before, place the paper or card on the floor and stand behind it. Take a deep breath and step onto it, and as you do this, imagine these changes are being uploaded into your mind. Imagine this is really happening and as you do, create in your mind's eye images of you doing these things over the next seven days. When you have done this fully, step off and imagine the week has already happened, and that now you have a week's experience under your belt. When you have fully done this, you really can see a week's worth of events having happened (which may highlight some pitfalls as well as benefits).

4. **Repeat the exercise in exactly the same way** for one month, three months and so on until you have a clear strategy on all six cards, *and* you have literally walked through and experienced it becoming reality.

5. **Now lay all the cards in a row in front of you like stepping stones.** After reading this instruction fully, step on to the first card and re-live that first day again. Then move straight on to the first week and relive that again, then the first month and so on. When you get to your last card, and you have changed all the things you need to change to achieve your goal, turn around and look back at how far you have come. See the old you standing way back, and send her the wisdom you have now from *experiencing* these 12 months of change. Talk to her out loud, tell her not to worry and that she can do it because you already have! Tell her

that as soon as she changes her mind, her body will start to change. Not at the same rate, but it will change definitely and purposefully into the healthy new shape you are now in the future. As you look back at all the changes you have made, do you like what you see?

6. **Close your eyes, and using the technique** you learnt on p.99 create a powerful, positive anchor for this feeling of certainty and achievement. Create absolute *faith* in your ability to achieve this, because you already have made the changes you wanted to make. Did you see those changes?

7. **You may wish to squeeze your fist at this point**, or press your tongue against the roof of your mouth (this is often used to aid focus). Or you can create your own physical movement that you can repeat anywhere, and at any time.

These six pieces of paper or card are now your strategy. You now have everything you need. But like all the best strategies, they are flexible. They can be improved and changed as you continue to develop new skills, and as positive thoughts become second nature. I recommend that you take a few minutes to lay the cards out and repeat this walk through *at least* once per week. The more you repeat it (with full-on emotion), the more entrenched it will become in your unconscious. Imagination is your reality. When you change in your mind, your body will change too.

I wish you joy for your journey. Please do join me on the *Think More Eat Less* Facebook page and keep in touch. Now you know the secret, share it by doing it. You have the power to passively teach and inspire others around you in a way that is more powerful than words.

Mabel's Journal

I thought it was funny that the goal-setting bit was at the end of the book, but now I've read it, I totally understand why. I've been making so many changes myself that I already have a strategy that I can work on, and it hasn't been dictated to me. I have developed it myself to suit me, so I know I am really in control. I've just been responding to what I've been learning, and as I made a conscious decision right from the start to DO this book rather than just read it, I certainly have done that! I have taken responsibility for what I can achieve: no more blaming it on anyone or anything else. That was a big thing for me.

As I did the exercise – walking through my six steps – it made me realize again, for the umpteenth time, how far I have come since I started this book and how much I am changing. I understand why Janet says to read it again. I will definitely do that – maybe not all of it right through, but I will go back and revisit the chapters when I want to have a re-charge. I've already read a couple of chapters twice, and it makes even more sense the second time!

The six steps were amazing. Actually _walking_ through my strategy, rather than just sitting down visualizing it, made it more real somehow. It reminded me of feeling closer to the slimmer me as I'm walking/running. Perhaps some psychic sense was at work, or perhaps I really have connected with the 'Infinite Intelligence' as Napoleon Hill puts it. Whatever it is, I'm much more instinctive and I really do have a definiteness of purpose. I feel I'm being guided, yet the funny thing is, I know I'm being guided

<u>by myself</u>. The 'me' inside who is confident, free, true and honest. I am finally listening to her, after years of shutting her away. She is forgiving too. She has forgiven the people who have dumped their SHIT on her over the years (though she still doesn't like some of them!). They probably just had other people's SHIT dumped on them. Not sure why I'm writing this bit, but it feels good because I know I'm now a SHIT-free zone!!

~~~~~~~~~~~~~~~~~~~~~

It's now nearly three weeks since I finished the Healthy Starter Plan and I just remembered to take my measurements. Shows how far I've come that I don't want or need to keep weighing myself! I have lost over 6 inches in total, almost a stone in weight and two dress sizes in just 11 weeks. That's bloody brilliant!!!!

~~~~~~~~~~~~~~~~~~~~~

It's now six weeks since I took my last measurements, and as expected, I have lost another 3 inches, and am definitely more toned up. My energy levels are fantastic! Still warm enough to do my workouts outside and I can now run for 20 minutes and walk for 10. I do a Zumba class most weeks too, just for fun!! Definitely on track for my December goal: might even get there sooner, but taking it one day at a time. My goal is a daily thing – on my mirror at the moment is: 'Do something good for your body (again) today.'

I stopped using the Daily Check Lists two weeks after the Healthy Starter Plan; I used them for a total of four weeks altogether, but now I don't need them anymore – I can. do it instantly in my head in seconds.

Each meal = 1 or no PINK (starchy stuff); minimum 2 GREEN (fruit and veg); 1 BLUE (high-quality fats and protein). Snacks = GREEN and BLUE only, no PINK.

REDS – occasionally in moderation.

~~~~~~~~~~~~~~~~~~~~~~~~~

It's now seven months since I started out at size 20. I am now a comfortable size 14 or 12. It's only four dress sizes, but I look and feel like a different person and really am not dieting at all, just looking after my body. The colour code system is totally ingrained into my thinking and I am so grateful that AT LAST I have put not only the misery of being fat behind me, I have also dumped so much emotional SHIT and feel totally liberated!

Three of my friends have now started the programme as they can see how much I have changed. I am quite excited for them!!! We are going to get together once a week to support each other, not just in terms of weight, but in all areas of our lives – like a 'positivity group' I guess!!

My cooking skills have improved no end and I'm actually spending less on food as I'm buying less meat and loads more veggies. My curry-making skills have become quite legendary and the girls have been round twice for a curry night in!!! Found a great tandoori chicken recipe online that I'm really pleased with. Simple things like chapatis instead of naan breads can save so many empty calories; I am constantly aware of not raising my blood sugar with refined rubbish that would just be turned into fat anyway! I've had to buy some new clothes, but I stuck to the cheap shops as I still have another size to go and I know now with absolute CERTAINTY that I will get there!

26 December

This year I got the BEST Christmas present EVER – I got my body back!!!

I arrived for Christmas dinner wearing a beautiful blue dress IN SIZE 12!!!! It wasn't too tight (even after dinner!!) and I didn't even need my Bridget Jones knickers!

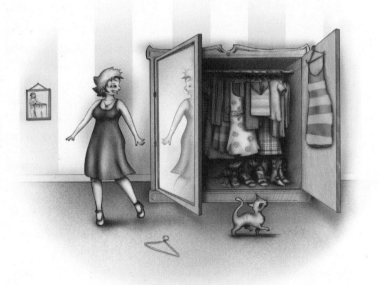

I was the talk of the day! Never had so many compliments, even from relatives who are less than polite. Of course, 'you know who' made a snidey comment, but you know what – that's just jealousy. It rolled off me like water off a duck's back – that's not my SHIT anymore!!!

For the first time in years, I am looking forward to New Year's Eve. This year has been life-changing for me. I am stronger emotionally, slimmer physically, so much fitter and healthier, more confident, more definite about what I want to achieve. I've also met new people who are like-minded and positive and I have a real purpose to my life now.

I give this journal as a gift, with genuine and sincere blessings. But you already know that being given a gift is one thing, you must choose to use it.

Love, Mabel x

USEFUL INFORMATION

For information on my seminars and workshops in your area, as well as one-to-one appointments, visit www. powertochange.me.uk.

For all of the free downloads to accompany the book, visit www.powertochange.me.uk. Click on the *Think More, Eat Less* link and enter the password 'Positive Attitude'.

RECOMMENDED READING

Think and Grow Rich – Napoleon Hill (Fawcett Books)

The Guide – Dr William Holden (Forecast Publishing)

Tapping For Life – Janet Thomson (Hay House Publishers)

Fats That Heal, Fats That Kill – Udo Erasmus (Alive Books)

INDEX

Index

'hitting the wall' 147, 163
and insulin resistance 145, 146,
    147
recording 223
and thyroid function 152, 153
types of 153–4, 158, 161–2,
    163–5

Facebook group xviii, 114, 117, 240
faith 19, 80–2, 108, 117, 240
fats
    cell size 157
    and exercise 147, 153–4, 158,
        160–2, 163, 165
    fatty acids 174–7, 178–82, 195,
        205, 210
    and hormones 132, 138, 139,
        141–2, 145–6
    low-fat dieting 187, 196
    and protein 184–5, 195
    see also BLUE group
fear 74, 89–90
feedback system 139, 145, 184, 197
feelings
    active 1–2, 3, 11
    and associations 24, 75, 77, 98,
        122
    desired feelings exercises 4–6,
        8–9
    see also anchors; emotions
fibre 136, 186, 210
food recording 67–8, 169–70, 187,
    208, 222–4
Frankl, Viktor 114–5
free will 35, 79
friends xviii, 113–4, 117
fructose 186, 189
fruit 189, 190, 199

glucose
    and burning fat 158, 159, 160,
        161–2
    food group 185, 186–7
    in ketosis 147–9, 163
    regulation 134, 138, 141–2, 145,
        146
gluten 133

Glycemic Index (GI) 175, 187–8
    and colour coding 189, 195, 196,
        220–1
goal setting 57, 66, 116–7, 235–40
Goodman, Morris 47–51, 71, 80–1,
    94, 109
GREEN group 189, 195, 198–200,
    220, 223
Green Peppercorn and Paprika
    Sauce 229
group support xviii, 113–4, 117, 240

Hay, Louise 3
Healthy Starter Pack 233
Healthy Starter Plan
    design 193–4, 207–10
    exercise regime 212
    portion sizes 199, 202, 204
    sample meals 210–2
high-protein, low-carb diets 148–9,
    159–60, 171–2, 183–4
Hill, Napoleon 18–20, 41, 51, 107–9,
    236
Holden, Will 116
hormones
    and exercise 146, 152, 161
    functions 75–6, 132, 138–42, 143
    and relaxation 150, 154, 160
hunter-gatherers 73, 117, 148,
    170–1
hydrochloric acid 183
hypnosis 43, 83, 84–8
    see also autosuggestion

iceberg, 'two minds' 22–3, 25–6,
    74, 98
imagination
    and reality 74, 89–90, 240
    setting anchors exercises 99–101,
        102–3
    using your 11, 19, 94–7, 104
incompetence, stages of 33, 34, 35
Infinite Intelligence 20, 41, 51–2,
    95, 115
insulin 138, 140–2, 148–9, 187
    insulin resistance (IR) 142––5,
        146–7

Index

internal voice 29
iodine 152–3

journal, progress xiii, xvi, 4, 90

ketosis 148, 149, 159
kidney function 183
knowledge 19, 30–1, 35–6, 118, 169

lean body mass (LBM) 146, 148,
    159, 161, 165
limitations, self-imposed 35, 52
Lipton, Bruce 3, 46, 47
liver function 133–7, 152, 208–9,
    233
luck 12, 41–2, 109
lunches 211, 224–5

Marconi, Guglielmo 39–40
Master Mind principle 20
measurements table xvi–xviii
meditation 154, 164
meridians 122–3, 124
metabolic rate 138, 152, 159, 165,
    172
mind
    mind-body connection 2–3, 122,
        207
    'two minds' iceberg 21–3, 25–7
Miracle Man *see* Goodman, Morris
mirror exercises 4–6, 98
monounsaturated fatty acids
    (MUFAs) 178, 179
muscle tissue
    and fat burning 146, 160–2, 165,
        184, 212
    ketosis 148, 149, 159

negative thinking
    anchors 98, 99–101
    and comfort eating 6, 8, 121–2
    manifesting events 11–2, 90,
        109
    versus positive 41–2, 115–6,
        123–4
    reject SHIT imprints 28–9, 31–2,
        43–5, 113, 115

TFT triangle technique 124–6
    as weeds 93–4
Neuro-Linguistic Programming (NLP)
    18
nocebo effect 47, 50
Novella, Dr Steven 78
nutrition course 67–8, 169

oestrogen 139–40, 152
Olson, Jeff 63
omega-3 176, 179, 180
omega-6 176, 179, 180
overeating
    causes 74–5, 76–8
    feedback mechanism 197–8
    reasons for 121
    self-harming 6–7
Overwhelmingly Positive Thoughts
    (OPT) 81–2, 97
oxytocin 140

pain 27, 77–8, 98, 102, 121–2
PCOS 143, 146
peak state 98–9, 100, 103
persistence 20, 42, 94
PINK group 189, 195, 200–2, 220,
    223
placebo effect 46–7
Plaice Fillet with Mushrooms and
    Pak Choi 230–1
pleasure 27, 74, 77
Polycystic Ovarian Syndrome (PCOS)
    143, 146
polyunsaturated fatty acids *see*
    essential fatty acids (EFAs)
portion sizes 196–8, 199, 201–2,
    203–4
positive thinking
    in childhood 43–4
    exercises and techniques 81–2,
        90, 102–3, 137, 240
    magnetic attraction 29, 113–4
    miracles demonstrating 48, 50–1,
        108, 109
    versus negativity 41–2, 115–6,
        123–4
steps to 116–8

250

Index

Index

triggers 74, 97–9
tryptophan 76

Udo's Oil 203, 210, 224, 225, 233
unconscious mind
  and Hill's principles 20, 41, 42
  protection instinct 73–4, 88
  self-hypnosis 82, 84
  stages of competence 33, 34, 35,
    222, 224
  'two minds' 21–2, 23, 25, 26
  and visualization 88–9
unsaturated fatty acids (UFAs) 174,
  176, 177–82

vegetables 136, 189–90, 198, 199,
  210
vibrational energy 40–1, 43, 51–2
visualizations
  audio download 102

in bed 11–2, 126
of goal 81–2, 96, 117
Morris Goodman's 48–9, 71
positive anchors exercises 102–3,
  137
unconscious effects 88–9, 90, 98

'walking through walls' 85–8
water 210
websites
  British Liver Trust 134
  IR test 145
  Miracle Man 51
  Udo Erasmus 181, 233
  see also Power To Change website
weight, charting your xvi–xviii
workshops 247

yoga 153, 154, 164

JOIN THE HAY HOUSE FAMILY

As the leading self-help, mind, body and spirit publisher in the UK, we'd like to welcome you to our family so that you can enjoy all the benefits our website has to offer.

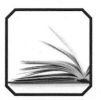

EXTRACTS from a selection of your favourite author titles

COMPETITIONS, PRIZES & SPECIAL OFFERS Win extracts, money off, downloads and so much more

LISTEN to a range of radio interviews and our latest audio publications

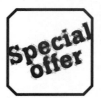

CELEBRATE YOUR BIRTHDAY An inspiring gift will be sent your way

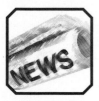

LATEST NEWS Keep up with the latest news from and about our authors

ATTEND OUR AUTHOR EVENTS Be the first to hear about our author events

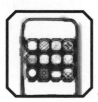

iPHONE APPS Download your favourite app for your iPhone

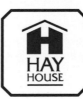

HAY HOUSE INFORMATION Ask us anything, all enquiries answered

join us online at **www.hayhouse.co.uk**

ABOUT THE AUTHOR

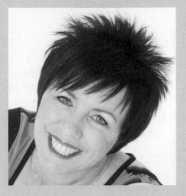 **Janet Thomson** is an outstanding Life Coach with a totally unique blend of skills and experience. She holds a Masters degree in Nutrition & Exercise Science, is an NLP (Neuro-linguistic Programming) Master Practitioner and Trainer, a TFT (Thought Field Therapy) Diagnostic Therapist and a registered Clinical Hypnotherapist. She combines these advanced skills with over 20 years of experience working with clients on an individual basis and in groups and seminars. This has firmly established her as a leader in the field of Personal Development and Achievement.

Janet is also a bestselling author, with her first book and fitness video *Fat To Flat* reaching No. 1 in the charts. She is an accomplished television presenter with appearances on GMTV and BBC1 and is now resident Health & Fitness Expert and Life Coach for ITV Central News. She regularly delivers seminars both for the general public and other instructors and coaches in the UK and abroad.

With a proven track record in the corporate sector, Janet was instrumental in setting up Rosemary Conley Diet & Fitness Clubs (RCDFC) and was personal consultant to Rosemary Conley, in addition to personally training over 100 RCDFC franchisees who went on to run successful businesses. Janet now runs her own Power To Change Private Coaching and Consultancy Practice. Those lucky enough to work with Janet enjoy great results and lasting change, making her one of the most sought after coaches in the UK.

www.powertochange.me.uk